CHRONIC PAIN

THE PATIENT AND FAMILY JOURNEY

ALAA ABD-ELSAYED, MD, MPH

The information provided in this book is based on best knowledge and currently available literature.

First edition, 2018.

ISBN: 9781791772710

Dedicated to

My patients who inspired me to edit this book.

My parents, my wife and my two beautiful kids,
Maro and George.

Alaa Abd-Elsayed, MD, MPH

TABLE OF CONTENTS

Contributing Authors

Thomas S. McDowell, MD, PhD, Associate Professor
Department of Anesthesiology
University of Wisconsin School of Medicine and Public
Health
Madison, Wisconsin, USA
Understanding Pain

Alaa Abd-Elsayed, MD, MPH
Medical Director, Pain Management
University of Wisconsin School of Medicine and Public
Health
Madison, Wisconsin, USA
Factors that Can Promote Chronic Pain

Nicholas Prayson, MD and Christine Zaky
Cleveland Clinic Foundation and University of
Pittsburgh, USA
Effect of Pain on Patient's and Family's Lives

Jay Karri, MD & Alaa Abd-Elsayed, MD, MPH
Department of Physical Medicine and Rehabilitation
Baylor College of Medicine
Houston, Texas, USA
Supporting Your Spouse in Chronic Pain

Matt Fischer, MD, MHA
Department of Anesthesiology
University of Wisconsin School of Medicine and Public
Health
Madison, Wisconsin, USA
Supporting Your Parents in Chronic Pain

Alaa Abd-Elsayed, MD, MPH
Medical Director, Pain Management
University of Wisconsin School of Medicine and Public
Health
Madison, Wisconsin, USA
Algorithm for Treating Chronic Pain

Tiffany M. Houdek, PT, OCS & Alaa Abd-Elsayed, MD,
MPH
Physical Therapy, University of Wisconsin School of
Medicine and Public Health
Madison, Wisconsin, USA
Non-Pharmological Therapies

Greta Nemergut, PharmD
University of Wisconsin Hospital and Clinics, UW Health
Madison, Wisconsin, USA
Nutrition and Pain

Greta Nemergut, PharmD
University of Wisconsin Hospital and Clinics, UW Health
Madison, Wisconsin, USA
Medications for Treating Chronic Pain

Larry Manders, MD, MBA, Raj Desai, MD, Alaa Abd-
Elsayed, MD, MPH
Pain Management
University of Wisconsin School of Medicine and Public
Health, Madison, Wisconsin, USA
Chronic Pain Procedures

Larry Manders, MD, MBA, Raj Desai, MD, Alaa Abd-
Elsayed, MD, MPH
Pain Management
University of Wisconsin School of Medicine and Public

Health, Madison, Wisconsin, USA
Advanced Pain Procedures

Larry Manders, MD, MBA & Alaa Abd-Elsayed, MD, MPH
Pain Management
University of Wisconsin School of Medicine and Public Health, Madison, Wisconsin, USA
Opioids and Their Hazards

Norann Richard, PhD
Psychology
CBI Health Centre, Canada
Treating Psychological Disorders Related to Pain

Larry Manders, MD, MBA & Alaa Abd-Elsayed, MD, MPH
Pain Management
University of Wisconsin School of Medicine and Public Health, Madison, Wisconsin, USA
Psychological Approaches for Treating Chronic Pain

Preface

Dear readers,

I was inspired to edit this book by my patients and their families. Some of my patients came to me after being seen in other pain clinics and in my opinion could have been treated in a better way. Not that other providers did not intend to treat them well but maybe lacked the knowledge to do so. In addition, I found that patients and their families need to learn more about the multidisciplinary approach for treating chronic pain, so they can understand the rationale behind our treatment decisions. In my practice, I worry not only about my patients but about their families too who can lose hope, develop depression, and have their lives revolve around chronic pain and their loved one who is suffering.

Patients show up to the pain clinic with many questions about their pain and its treatment; this book will provide chronic pain patients with essential information on their pain and its management. In addition, since the psychological and social issues arising from pain impact patient's spouses, children, and other family members, it is crucial that these populations also learn about chronic pain to be able to work with their loved ones combatting chronic pain. I cannot stress enough the importance of family support to help chronic pain patients in their treatment journey.

I hope this book will help patients and their families go through the pain management journey with knowledge and confidence. While chronic pain is a challenging condition, it can be controlled by several means including non-pharmacological, pharmacological, psychological, and interventional techniques.

My message from this book to all patients and their loved ones: stay strong and positive. We have several ways to treat pain and we will do our best to help you gain your life back. I cannot tell you how many times we turned patients' lives from depression to happiness, from thinking it is the end to thinking this is the beginning, from being inactive to be able to travel all around the world. Do not let pain win, YOU are the winner.

Editor

Alaa Abd-Elsayed, MD, MPH

UNDERSTANDING PAIN

Introduction

Our ability to sense acute pain helps us protect our bodies from potentially harmful environmental dangers. Touching the tip of a sharp knife in a drawer or a hot pan on the stove, elicits pain that tells us we should withdraw our hand and care for our injury. Individuals with diminished pain sensation may develop wounds that are ignored, get infected and may require amputation (e.g. those with diabetic neuropathy), or in rare cases, they may suffer from self-mutilation (individuals with congenital insensitivity to pain). In this way we can think of acute pain as being beneficial to our health, which is why it is sometimes referred to as "physiological pain" [1-3].

Sometimes, however, pain is not protective. It may persist beyond an initial injury, even after that injury has been treated, and can become an annoyance (think paper cut). This type of pain often goes away as the injury heals, but sometimes acute pain can persist and develop into chronic pain. More than an annoyance, chronic pain can be debilitating and significantly impact our lives. Chronic pain is sometimes called "pathological pain", implying that the pain itself has become a disease that needs to be treated [1-3].

Much of the information in this chapter describes what we know about physiological pain. This chapter will discuss the structure and function of the peripheral nerves involved in pain sensation and transmission, how pain transmission is regulated in the spinal cord, and how some of the drugs we take for the treatment of pain work. Less is known about the mechanisms of chronic pathological pain, and to explain what we do know about it requires a knowledge of neurobiology that is beyond the scope of this chapter to review. However, this chapter includes some general information about the development of peripheral and central sensitization, which can explain some forms of chronic pain.

Structure of Primary Nociceptive Neurons

Specialized neurons in our body sense pain. They are called primary nociceptive neurons, or primary nociceptors. Like other sensory neurons, such as those that sense things like light touch, temperature, and vibration, primary nociceptors are part of the peripheral nervous system (the spinal cord and brain comprise the central nervous system). The cell bodies of sensory neurons contain important structures like the nucleus and reside in ganglia (a ganglion is a structure that contains multiple cell bodies) which each contain perhaps tens of thousands of individual sensory neuron cell bodies. The cell bodies of neurons that innervate the head reside in ganglia near the brain. The cell bodies of neurons that innervate the rest of the body reside in ganglia near the back (dorsum) of the spinal cord where sensory nerve roots enter and are called dorsal root ganglia. There are 31 pairs of dorsal root ganglia in the human body [1].

The other main part of a sensory neuron is the axon. The axon is basically a cable that neurons use to transmit electrical information from one location in the body to another. Actually, all sensory neurons can be described as having two axons, one peripheral branch that receives sensory information from the body and sends it to the cell body, and one central branch that relays that information from the cell body to the central nervous system. Sensory neurons that innervate the toe are among the longest cells in the body. Their peripheral axons start in the toe and run up the leg to the cell body that resides in a dorsal root ganglion near the spine.

Their central axons then extend from the cell body to the base of the spinal cord. That makes these cells several feet long [1]. Peripheral nerves like the sciatic nerve contain a number of sensory nerve axons (peripheral branches), but not all of these axons are the same. They vary by size (cross-sectional diameter) and by the degree of myelination. Myelin is a sheath formed when other cells that reside along the axon (Schwann cells) wrap around the neuronal axon. This provides electrical insulation to the axon. Large axons with the most myelin transmit electrical signals the fastest. These axons are associated with sensory neurons that provide information about the positions of your body parts in space; this information needs to be transmitted to the brain quickly, so our movements can be coordinated, and we don't fall over. Primary nociceptors, on the other hand, have the smallest axons, with little or no myelin, and thus are among the slowest conducting axons of all sensory neurons. Using the standard classification scheme, nociceptor axons are either C-fibers (small axon, no myelin) or Aδ-fibers (small axon, thinly myelinated). As you might expect, Aδ- fibers have a slightly faster conduction velocity than C-fibers but are still slow compared to most other types of sensory nerve axons. Because of their faster transmission, Aδ-fiber nociceptors are thought to be responsible for "first" or "fast" pain that is well localized, sharp, stabbing, or pricking. Unmyelinated C-fiber nociceptors are thought to transmit "second" or "slow" pain that is often poorly localized and described as dull, burning, or aching [1-3].

Function of Primary Nociceptive Neurons

How do painful (noxious) physical stimuli like a pinch, a cut, or a burn injury activate, or "turn on", primary nociceptors? First let's talk about what it means to activate a sensory neuron. All neurons, including primary nociceptors, are negatively charged at rest. One way of thinking about it is that neurons have fewer positively charged ions inside them than there are in the fluid that surrounds them (negatively charged ions are less important for this discussion). When we talk about neurons being activated, we talk about them "spiking" or "firing". That just means that they quickly and briefly switch their negative charge to a positive charge. Whenever a neuron's charge gets less negative, even just by a little bit, it is called a depolarization. During this special "spike", however, the depolarization is about as big as they come, though it lasts for just a few milliseconds before the neuron goes back to having its normal negative charge. This depolarizing spike is called an action potential.

Action potentials are generated primarily by the rapid opening and closing of sodium channels. Sodium channels are proteins embedded in the membranes of neurons that let positively charged sodium ions flow into the cell when they are open. Even though they only open for a few milliseconds before they close, enough sodium ions pass through the open channels and enter the neuron that it causes the massive depolarization that creates an action potential. If you block sodium channels from opening right where a neuron is being stimulated, you will prevent action potentials from forming and you will keep the neuron from being activated. If you block sodium channels in the nerve axon (i.e., in the peripheral nerves that carry sensory neuron axons) you can keep action potentials from traveling up the axon to the central nervous system. It turns out that sodium channels are easily and completely blocked by local anesthetics. So, when you get a "numbing injection" of a local anesthetic before a procedure at the dentist or at the hospital, or wear a lidocaine patch, or get a labor epidural for childbirth, you don't feel pain because the local anesthetic is blocking the sodium channels in the primary nociceptors. Action potentials are thus prevented from reaching the central nervous system, which otherwise would lead you to become aware of the pain.

Sodium channels not only cause the depolarization of the action potential, they are also triggered to open by depolarization. This ends up creating a positive feedback cycle that keeps action potentials traveling all the way from one end of a neuron to the other. Without it, a depolarization (even a large one like an action potential) would gradually die out over a short distance due to resistance to ion flow in the axon. In the peripheral terminals of primary nociceptors, small depolarizations are generated when the neuron detects a painful stimulus.

These depolarizations are much smaller than the depolarization of an action potential, but they can trigger sodium channels to open. Once the sodium channels open, they produce an action potential that signals neuronal activation in response to the painful stimulus. How does a physical stimulus like painful, burning heat get turned into a depolarization in a neuron? It is all due to a specialized protein with a strange name, TRPV1, which is found exclusively on heat-sensitive primary nociceptors. TRPV1 is an ion channel like the sodium channel, but instead of opening in response to depolarization, it opens in response to noxious heat. So, when the nerve endings in our finger, for example, are heated to temperatures that we sense as painful (> 43°C), the TRPV1 channel opens. Positively charged then enter the neuron, causing a small depolarization, which opens sodium channels, generating action potentials which travel along the axon to the central nervous system, and that's how we can tell that our finger is getting burned [1-5].

The other interesting part of this story is that noxious heat is not the only thing that causes the TRPV1 channel to open. It also opens in the presence of capsaicin, a chemical produced by hot peppers that is, in fact, the reason that peppers taste hot. It is also the active ingredient in pepper spray. That burning sensation you feel in your mouth when you bite into a jalapeno pepper comes from the capsaicin activating TRPV1. You are activating the same nociceptors with the capsaicin that you would with noxious heat, and the nociceptors can't tell the difference. That's why the pain of the pepper is described as a burning pain. But capsaicin isn't all bad. At lower doses capsaicin creams and patches can be applied to the skin to treat pain.

That's because continuous capsaicin application can actually cause TRPV1 and the nociceptors it activates to become desensitized, not only to noxious heat but to other types of pain as well, so they become much less likely to respond to a painful stimulus.

Persistent Pain and Primary Nociceptors

Unfortunately, physiological pain sometimes becomes persistent. This can be due to changes in the primary nociceptors that are generally referred to as peripheral sensitization. There are two types of persistent pain caused by sensitization of the primary nociceptor: inflammatory pain and neuropathic pain. As its name suggests, inflammatory pain is due to tissue inflammation that results from a local injury, such as a burn, a cut, or a crush injury.

Inflammation can be recognized by localized swelling, redness, and heat after an injury. These changes are mediated by chemical mediators released by damaged cells in the injured tissue and by immune cells that migrate to the site of injury to help prevent infection. Unfortunately, many of these chemical mediators also act on the primary nociceptor nerve endings and can either directly activate them or make them more sensitive so they fire more action potentials for a given stimulus. This is referred to as primary hyperalgesia [1-3]. The so-called non- steroidal anti-inflammatory drugs (NSAIDs) like ibuprofen can help control inflammatory pain directly by reducing inflammation and decreasing the production of pain-inducing chemical mediators. Specifically, NSAIDs block the activity of an enzyme called cyclooxygenase. This enzyme responds to injury by producing mediators (prostaglandins and leukotrienes), that not only contribute to inflammation but also sensitize nociceptors. Thus, blocking the activity of this enzyme reduces inflammatory pain.

The other type of persistent pain that can be due to sensitization of primary nociceptors is called neuropathic pain. Peripheral neuropathic pain (as opposed to central neuropathic pain which is defined as pain initiated or caused by a primary lesion in the central nervous system "e.g. stroke") arises after either physical damage or some type of metabolic insult to peripheral nociceptors. Physical damage to primary nociceptors includes traumatic injuries, post-surgical changes, and pinched nerves. Metabolic insults include damage due to diabetes, herpes zoster, and some types of chemotherapy. Unlike inflammatory pain, neuropathic pain is more difficult to treat and is more likely to become chronic [1-4].

Pain Transmission in the Spinal Cord

The spinal cord can be divided into ten layers, or laminae, based on their appearance and cell content. The posterior part of the spinal cord, called the dorsal horn, is comprised of six laminae and is where all sensory information enters. Primary nociceptors send their central axons into the two most dorsal layers, lamina I and lamina II, where they make contact with the cells residing there. Laminae I and II collectively are referred to collectively as the superficial dorsal horn. Lamina I contains second-order nociceptor cell bodies which send their axons directly up to higher brain centers, like the thalamus and cortex, the parts of our central nervous system that allow us to perceive pain. Also present in lamina I are a large number of interneurons, which are neurons whose axons do not leave the dorsal horn (they are "internal" to the dorsal horn). Interneurons just make contact with other neurons within the spinal cord. Lamina II contains only the cell bodies of interneurons. Some interneurons are excitatory, meaning they can activate other neurons they make contact with. Other interneurons are inhibitory, meaning they can inhibit the activity of other neurons. As such, when the central axons of primary nociceptors enter the superficial dorsal horn, they may make contact with second- order nociceptors in lamina I directly, or they may contact either excitatory or inhibitory interneurons first, which then may contact second-order nociceptors in lamina I, for example, either directly or through even more interneurons.

Under normal circumstances there is a balance between these excitatory and inhibitory forces so that acute physiological pain is sensed and transmitted faithfully in the central nervous system for the health and safety of the individual without allowing extreme or chronic pathological pain to develop or persist [2,5,6,7].

The only other group of cells that primary nociceptors are known to make contact with are referred to as wide dynamic range (WDR) neurons. These neurons are found deeper in the dorsal horn (laminae III-VI). Unlike the second-order nociceptors in lamina I which only receive input about painful stimuli, WDR neurons receive input from both primary nociceptors and non- nociceptive neurons, such as those that transmit light touch. That's how they get their name, because they respond to a wide range of stimuli. WDR neurons may represent a key element of the neuronal circuit that was proposed by Patrick Wall and

Ronald Melzack over 50 years ago to explain their gate control theory of pain. Although WDR neurons had not been identified at that time, these investigators conceived of a neuron that received input from both nociceptors and non-nociceptors. In their model, when a non-nociceptive neuron contacting a WDR neuron is activated, it causes an inhibitory interneuron to inhibit or "close the gate" on input from a primary nociceptor to the WDR neuron. This circuit could explain the observation that pain can sometimes be diminished by holding or rubbing the affected area because these actions activate non-nociceptive neurons that would inhibit the pain signal at the WDR neuron [2,5,7].

The final modulatory influence on the pain signal in the spinal cord actually comes from the brain. Although we think of pain information as traveling "up" from the periphery to the brain, the brain also sends information "down" to the spinal dorsal horn via axons of specialized brain neurons along what are called descending pathways. These descending pathways influence pain transmission even more, adding both inhibitory and excitatory influences on an already highly modulated pain signal [7].

Opioids are some of the most widely used and effective medications we have to reduce pain. Our own body produces opioids (these are called endogenous opioids) that contribute to the normal inhibition of pain transmission in both the spinal dorsal horn and through descending pathways as discussed above. Exogenous opioid medications given to treat pain exploit and enhance these endogenous systems. Opioids mostly act at three different parts of the pain pathway. They inhibit primary nociceptors from activating their neuronal targets in the dorsal horn. They also decrease the excitability of second-order nociceptors i the dorsal horn, so they are less likely to respond to activating sign from primary nociceptors. Finally, they also act in the brain, specifi increasing the activity of inhibitory descending pathways, thus lea further suppression of the pain signal [6]. However, opioids p wide range of side effects which are discussed in another chapter. In addition, opioids represent the biggest killer in the USA. Therefore, their use must be implemented with caution and only for certain patients.

Other more popular medications used for treating acute and chronic pain include antiseizure medications and antidepressants among other agents (discussed in more details in a different chapter).

Central Sensitization of Pain

Sometimes acute, physiological pain leads to the development of chronic, pathological pain. As mentioned above, primary nociceptors can become sensitized during tissue inflammation or after a traumatic or metabolic insult. This peripheral sensitization in the primary nociceptors can sometimes be the root cause of chronic pain, but increased activity of primary nociceptors can also induce changes in dorsal horn neurons that lead to what is called central sensitization.

How does central sensitization take place? There have been many studies implicating a variety of chemicals and receptors in the development of central sensitization. Without going into too much detail, there are three main ways that central sensitization is thought to occur. One is that a loss of the normal inhibitory influences in the dorsal horn simply leads to more excitatory activity in the pain pathway. This could occur either through a decrease in inhibitory interneuron function and/or a decrease in the strength of descending inhibitory signals from the brain [1,2].

ʰanism to explain central sensitization is increased ᵈ-order nociceptors in the dorsal horn. Remember of primary nociceptors enter the dorsal horn of make contact with a number of different cell types ,econd-order nociceptors and WDR neurons. Activity (action potentials) in the primary nociceptors normally crosses over to the other neurons, in turn activating them in a proportional manner according to the other excitatory and inhibitory influences normally active in the dorsal horn. When there is a lot of activity in the primary nociceptors (e.g., pain intensity is great or there is peripheral sensitization), it causes activation of a special protein, called the NMDA receptor, in second-order nociceptors and WDR neurons. Under normal conditions the NMDA receptor does nothing, but when activated it induces changes in neurons that increase their responsiveness to normal stimuli. Basically, the second-order nociceptors become hyperexcitable and thus amplify the pain signal coming from the primary nociceptors. A similar phenomenon occurs in areas of the brain that are involved in memory formation, where it is called long-term potentiation. WDR neurons demonstrate a unique pattern of hyperexcitability known as wind-up [1,2,7].

The third mechanism explaining central sensitization is more complex, and somewhat surprising. One of the cardinal signs of experimental central sensitization is that normally innocuous mechanical stimulation (e.g., light touch, stroking) in areas surrounding the original site of pain or injury now becomes painful. This is referred to as secondary hyperalgesia, as opposed to primary hyperalgesia which was discussed earlier. In this situation, sensory fibers that normally carry innocuous stimuli make new, or stronger, contacts with pain-sensitive neurons in the spinal cord, thus shifting their normal pattern of transmission to pain circuits so that activation of these neurons is perceived as pain in the brain. Recall that WDR neurons are known to have inputs from both primary nociceptors and non-nociceptive neurons, and thus may contribute to this secondary hyperalgesia. It is likely that a similar mechanism probably also explains the development of allodynia seen with neuropathic pain. Allodynia is the sensation of pain from normally innocuous (non-painful) stimuli. Unlike secondary hyperalgesia, however, allodynia is not limited to the area surrounding a previously injured or painful site [1,2].

Summary

- Acute pain is sometimes called physiological pain. Because it alerts us to real or potential environmental dangers, it is generally viewed as being beneficial to our health. When pain persists and becomes chronic, it is no longer beneficial. It is sometimes called pathological pain, implying that pain itself is a disease that needs to be treated.

- We sense painful stimuli because we have highly specialized sensory neurons called primary nociceptive neurons that only respond to painful stimuli like cuts or noxious heat. The cell bodies of primary nociceptors reside in ganglia along with the cell bodies of other sensory neurons near the central nervous system. They have peripheral axons that transmit information about painful stimuli from tissues to the cell body, and central axons that then transmit that information from the cell body directly to the central nervous system (brain or spinal cord).

- The peripheral axons of primary nociceptors, which run in peripheral nerves, are among the smallest of all sensory axons. C-fiber axons have no myelin sheath and thus have very slow conduction velocities. Aδ-fiber axons are thinly myelinated and so have slightly faster conduction velocities than C-fiber axons. Aδ-fiber nociceptors are thought to be responsible for "first" or "fast" pain that is well localized, sharp, stabbing, or pricking. C-fiber nociceptors are thought to transmit "second" or "slow" pain that is often poorly localized and described as a dull, burning, or aching pain.

- Sodium channels, present in all neurons, are responsible for generating action potentials that indicate a neuron has been activated. Action potentials travel down an axon from one end of the neuron to the other without losing strength. Local anesthetics like lidocaine block sodium channels, which blocks action potential formation and/or transmission and thus prevents pain signals generated by primary nociceptors from reaching the central nervous system, so pain is not perceived.

- Capsaicin, the active ingredient in hot peppers, activates heat-sensitive primary nociceptor nerve endings by causing a heat-sensitive ion channel called TRPV1 to open. That's why peppers leave you with a burning pain. Capsaicin can also cause desensitization of nociceptors after prolonged application, so it is sometimes used as a cream or patch on the skin to treat chronic pain.

- Sometimes acute pain can become persistent. In primary nociceptors, this can be either inflammatory or neuropathic in nature. In inflammatory pain, chemical mediators released from injured tissue or immune cells can directly activate or increase the sensitivity of primary nociceptive nerve endings. NSAIDs can be used to treat this pain as they block the cyclooxygenase enzyme that makes some of the mediators that cause sensitization. Neuropathic pain can be due to physical nerve injury or metabolic insults like chemotherapy or diabetes.

- The central axons of primary nociceptive neurons make contact primarily with cells in the first two layers of the dorsal horn of the spinal cord, known as the superficial dorsal horn. Cells in these layers include second-order nociceptors, as well as both excitatory and inhibitory interneurons which modulate the pain signal. Primary nociceptors also contact wide dynamic range (WDR) neurons in deeper layers of the dorsal horn. WDR neurons also receive input from non-nociceptive neurons, such as those that respond to light touch. Descending fibers, which are axons of neurons from higher brain centers, are so called because they descend from the brain and make contact with many of the cells in the dorsal horn to modulate transmission of the pain signal.

- Opioids work on several levels in the spinal cord. They inhibit primary nociceptors from activating their neuronal targets in the dorsal horn. They also decrease the excitability of second-order nociceptors in the dorsal horn, so they are less likely to respond to activating signals from primary nociceptors. In addition, they increase the activity of inhibitory descending pathways from the brain. They have to be used carefully due to their wide range of side effects that leads to significant morbidity and mortality.

- Like peripheral nociceptors, pain-sensitive neurons in the spinal dorsal horn can become hyperexcitable, a phenomenon known as central sensitization. There are three main ways for this to develop. First, there can be a loss of normal inhibition, either through a decrease in inhibitory interneuron function and/or a decrease in the strength of descending inhibitory signals from the brain. Second, there can be an increase in excitability of second- order nociceptors. This is mediated by activation of a special protein, called the NMDA receptor, during intense activity from primary nociceptors. Third, neurons that normally sense innocuous stimuli like light touch can make new, or stronger, contacts with pain- sensitive neurons in the spinal cord so activation of these neurons is perceived as pain. This is responsible for secondary hyperalgesia surrounding an area of primary hyperalgesia. A similar mechanism probably explains the development of allodynia, the sensation of pain from normally innocuous stimuli.

References

1.Ringkamp M et al. Peripheral mechanisms of cutaneous nociception. In: McMahon SB, Koltzenburg M, Tracey I, Turk DC, editors. Wall and Melzack's Textbook of pain, 6th ed. Philadelphia: Saunders; 2013. p. 1-30.

2. Basbaum AI et al. Cellular and molecular mechanisms of pain. Cell. 2009; 139:267-84.

3. Dubin AE, et al. Nociceptors: the sensors of the pain pathway. J Clin Invest. 2010; 120:3760-72.

4. Gold MS. Molecular biology of sensory transduction. In: McMahon SB, Koltzenburg M, Tracey I, Turk DC, editors. Wall and Melzack's Textbook of pain, 6th ed. Philadelphia: Saunders; 2013. p. 31-47.

5. Benarroch EE. Dorsal horn circuitry: Complexity and implications for mechanisms of neuropathic pain. Neurology 2016; 86:1060-9.

6. Sorkin LS, et al. Spinal pharmacology of nociceptive transmission. In: McMahon SB, Koltzenburg M, Tracey I, Turk DC, editors. Wall and Melzack's Textbook of pain, 6th ed. Philadelphia: Saunders; 2013. p. 375-401.

7. Todd AJ, et al. Neuroanatomical substrates of spinal nociception. In: McMahon SB, Koltzenburg M, Tracey I, Turk DC, editors. Wall and Melzack's Textbook of pain, 6th ed. Philadelphia: Saunders; 2013. p. 77-93.

FACTORS THAT CAN PROMOTE CHRONIC PAIN

Introduction

There are several factors that can promote and increase the severity of chronic pain such as life stressors in general, work stressors, marriage problems, anxiety, depression, family stressors and more. It is very important during the course of treating chronic pain to manage these stressors otherwise treating chronic pain can be difficult if not impossible. While health care providers diligently to treat chronic pain using all available tools, in addition to psychological support, it is very crucial that the patient identify stressors in their life and try to overcome them the best they can. The presence of stressors can completely reduce the efficacy of all management the patient receives. Reducing life stressors sometimes requires not only patient effort but also the support of family, friends and colleagues support.

This chapter will discuss the most important stressors a patient with chronic pain can encounter. Some of these stressors may be unrecognizable to the patient, which is why it is important to identify both internal and external stressors and work with care providers on reducing them.

1- Psychological factors

It is very important to understand the biopsychosocial view to explain and describe chronic pain. This model describes the physical, pathological, social and psychological variables that contribute to chronic pain [1].

A. Patient beliefs

Patient beliefs play an important role on how patients perceive their pain, react to their pain, and set their expectations for pain management. For example, a patient's fear of moving a painful joint might increase his/her pain which leads to lack of participation in physical therapy, development of joint stiffness, and decreases the ability to move the joint. This in turn decreases the patient's ability to work and socialize. Over time these changes may lead to depression and anxiety due to the inability to perform simple activities causing isolation.

B. Self-efficacy

The self-efficacy expectation is defined as a personal conviction that one can successfully perform certain required behaviors in a given situation. Patients should work on performing activities without avoiding the use the painful joint or limb. This will make a patient more engaged in physical therapy which in turn will improve their condition. In addition, this will allow the patient to be more able to perform daily activities and socialize. This will likely result in the patient being less liable to depression, anxiety and other psychological conditions.

C. Disability

It has been reported that the presence of psychological comorbidities in chronic pain patient can promote disability.

In context of the aforementioned psychological factors, patient that work to be more active and functional despite their pain are less likely to be subjected to a sedentary life, additional pain, psychological and/or social problems, and disability. It is the patient's choice to move one way or another. While easier said than done, I would like patients to put forth the effort to move in a healthier direction. Though it will certainly require familial support and great willpower, the positive ending makes it all worth it. On the other hand, a sedentary lifestyle poses additional challenges to managing pain and returning to the lifestyle the patient has become accustomed to prior to their chronic pain.

2- Patient related factors

A. Expression of pain

The expression of pain is different among different cultures and different patients. Individuals surrounding the patient need to be aware of this, as some patients may express severe pain that may be out of proportion to radiographic and examination findings. This is due to their own individual threshold for feeling pain and their strong expression. Providers and family members may think the patient is exaggerating which is entirely possible, but we need to keep in mind that patients feel and express pain differently [2].

B. Using traditional remedies and prayer.

Using remedies and prayer may delay the start of medical treatment and in turn worsen the pain resulting in making it harder to treat later on. Prayer is important if the patient believes in its power, but it is not enough to treat chronic pain. Seeking medical advice is very important early on to allow for early and effective management of chronic pain.

C. Language barriers.

Language barriers can lead to ineffective communication with providers. Patients may not be able to accurately express their pain and providers may fail to appreciate the severity of pain. Communication is very important to accurately describe the pain and help providers to offer effective treatment. In addition, effective communication will help patients understand and follow a treatment plan leading to quicker recovery.

3- Providers' factors

Providers can differ in the way they approach and treat pain. They also differ on how they communicate with the patient. It is important to be treated by a knowledgeable provider that the patient trusts. The

23

physician-patient relationship is a very important factor in the success of the treatment plan.

4- Health system factors

There are several factors related to health care systems that can make treatment difficult. Some of the barriers existing in health systems include access and insurance coverage.

5- Life stressors

We encounter several stressors in our life. Stressors in the work place, stressors in marriage, stressors within the family, stressors related to other comorbidities, financial stressors, and more. A patient has to identify what stressors exist in their life and try their best to overcome them. Patients may be able to accomplish this on their own or with the help of professionals through counseling. Sometimes patients will not be able to overcome certain stressors and in this case, patients need to learn coping with those stressors to reduce their effects. There are several strategies to overcome or control stressors and reduce their negative effects on both the patients and their health.

Often, when I ask my patients what exacerbates or worsens their pain, they respond, "stress." Stress is common trigger for several pain conditions, which is why it is imperative to learn to cope with pain and stressors; coping with chronic pain and stressors falls under two big categories: active coping and passive coping. Active coping includes problem solving, regulation of emotion, focusing attention on the emotional response aroused by the stressor, and maintaining a positive attitude. Active coping is associated with less pain, less depression and less disability. Passive coping includes simple avoidance and escape, which leads to more pain, more depression, and greater functional impairment [3,4].

Summary

There are several factors that can worsen chronic pain and can represent a barrier to effective treatment. Those factors can be internal (patient related) or external. It is important to identify these stressors and either eliminate them or learn to cope with them to reduce their effect on pain and general well-being. It can be difficult for patients to identify these stressors, which is where professional assistance may be necessary to identify stressors and provide solutions to manage them.

References

1. Turk, D. C. et al. Chronic pain: A biobehavioral perspective. In R. J. Gatchel & D. C. Turk (Eds.), Psychosocial factors in pain: Critical perspectives (p. 18– 34). 1999, New York: Guilford Press.

2. Cornally N, et al. Chronic Pain: The Help-Seeking Behavior, Attitudes, and Beliefs of Older Adults Living in the Community. Pain Management Nursing 2011; 12: 206-217.

3. Ersek M, et al. Kemp CA. Use of the chronic pain coping inventory to assess older adults' pain coping strategies. J Pain. 2006; 7:833–842.

4. Büssing A, et al. Adaptive coping and spirituality as a resource in cancer patients. Breast Care. 2007; 2:195–202.

EFFECT OF PAIN ON PATIENT'S AND FAMILY'S LIVES

Introduction

Chronic pain is a leading public health issue in the United States. The National Center for Health Statistics conducted a nationwide questionnaire that estimated around 1 in 5 adults across the country suffer from chronic pain and almost half of these affected adults, or about 20 million people, reported that their pain limited life or work activities on most days.

Although chronic pain can afflict any type of person, it seems that in certain populations, chronic pain is more prevalent. According to the Center for Disease Control, those more likely to experience chronic pain include women, elderly people, those without a college degree, previously employed adults, those with low socioeconomic status, and those living in more rural settings [1]. Chronic pain sufferers are more likely to be a female, without a college degree, in fair or poor health, be obese, and have depressive symptoms.

Though various subgroups or attributes seem to be associated with an increased risk of chronic pain prevalence, chronic pain is quite universal in its presence. The implications of chronic pain are far reaching from a societal perspective, as well as from the perspective of the individual suffering from chronic pain. Given the prevalence of chronic pain, it is important to appreciate the impact it has upon many facets of a chronic pain sufferers' life, including activity, social life, sleep, work, and disability. Awareness of the implications chronic pain may have on these facets can help patients, caregivers, and care providers to attend to the patient's needs more holistically, in order to optimize their quality of life, and to consider the obstacles chronic pain patients may face. Additionally, being cognizant of some of the ways chronic pain impacts the lives of family and loved ones is also important.

Daily Function

The influence of chronic pain on daily function has been difficult to fully quantify. In order to best appreciate such a topic, we should explain what we mean by "daily function". Chronic pain can limit one's ability to partake in activities associated with daily life such as walking, daily chores, and other basic physical activities. Since pain is something that cannot be objectively measured, understanding the impact chronic pain has on physical activity is not a simple task.

Logically, one might assume that those with chronic pain would be less active in order to minimize pain. Many researchers have investigated this very idea with the hope of identifying just how limiting chronic pin can be upon daily physical function. One significant questionnaire of chronic pain sufferers conducted in Olmstead County, Minnesota showed that 26% of these people felt that chronic pain significantly interfered with their general activity and 25% believed that it impacted their ability to walk [2]. In other words, about a quarter of people reported an inability to function in their normal daily activities. A comprehensive review of the literature performed by Maria Dueñas and colleagues indicated that many studies suggest that chronic pain, whether it be lower back pain or fibromyalgia, can cause the pain sufferer to have decreased ability to perform daily tasks and activities [3]. Such findings should not be ignored, but it is important to note that such findings were not universal.

Questionnaires, such as the one mentioned earlier that was performed in Olmstead County, often play a large role in research studies examining the impact of chronic pain on daily function. Such studies often focus on one's perception of how chronic pain impacts daily living, rather than its actual impact. Importantly, such self-perceptions may not ultimately be accurate. In other words, someone with chronic pain may overestimate the impact chronic pain has on daily function.

Interestingly, some other studies have indicated that there is no clear difference in daily physical activity in those with chronic pain compared to those without chronic pain [3,4]. Rita J. van den Berg-Emons and colleagues, using accelerometer-based monitoring, determined that there was little to no difference in the length of activity between those with chronic pain and those without chronic pain [4]. These negative studies may offer some hope for chronic pain sufferers because they suggest that those suffering from chronic pain can be quite resilient in spite of their perceived limitations. Recognizing that one can participate in daily activities in a similar fashion to those without chronic pain, despite one's chronic pain, can be motivational.

It is crucial that one also understands how frequent mental health challenges and chronic pain can coincide. Chronic pain sufferers often struggle with mental health difficulties. It was identified that about a third of individuals with chronic spinal pain also had mental health disorders, such as anxiety, depression, and substance abuse difficulties. If one is suffering from any of these conditions, then one must address these in conjunction with attempting to manage his or her chronic pain. The goal is improved function and health status.

One must also not ignore the other health issues that such individuals face. The impact chronic pain has upon an individual should be assessed on an individual basis, while considering a number of variables. Such variables include, one's coping strategies, other stressors, physical health, cause of pain, psychological well-being, severity of pain, physical activity, interests and more. It has been found that an individual's belief in his or her own ability to manage chronic pain has a significant impact upon his or her ability to minimize disability [5]. This is important because it demonstrates that there are other areas of one's life that one can try to improve upon that may ultimately result in improved function, despite dealing with chronic pain.

Logically speaking, a physically healthy individual with low work and home stress, good social support, and strong coping strategies will likely report that his or her chronic pain does not negatively impact his or her functional life as much as someone who has many other medical conditions, poor coping strategies, high levels of social or work-related stress and poor support. As a result, one can reflect on how these factors may be affecting one's own life and consequently may be influencing how he or she perceives pain. It is just as important to focus on improving these factors such as developing supportive relationships, honing coping strategies and reducing stress to improve the patient's ability to manage chronic pain. There are many ways to do this and no clear blue print for every person. Some examples may include, yoga, meditation, exercise, socializing, support groups, or connecting with nature. It is up to the individual to strive to have an open mind and attempt to find and develop the strategies that work for them.

Activities

Someone suffering from chronic pain may become fearful of participating in activities that she or he used to enjoy. These fears may manifest in many ways: one will not be able to move with the same enthusiasm, fear of frustration due to an inability to complete a certain activity, and fear of losing interest. However, daily movement does not need to and should not stop because of chronic pain! Turk and Winter offered a strategy to handling this concern by focusing on moving "smarter, not harder" [6]. This strategy begins by learning the range of motion that causes the least pain in your body, and then figuring out how you can complete your daily activities within that range. You want to learn how to use your muscles efficiently and not subject them to strenuous activity that could possibly tear them and cause further pain. But one should not avoid painful activity or movements to the detriment of his or her physical health and thereby increase one's risk for injury. For example, patients should be aware that extreme forms of favoring one part of the body over time, can ultimately lead to wear and tear in other areas that are now being used in unusual and perhaps unnatural ways (e.g. leaning more on the left lower extremity due to pain in the right knee, over time the left side may hurt too due to overuse). This process can potentially lead to injury and additional pain. One might question how he or she can safely manage this balancing act. Physical therapy experts can be useful in helping one identify safe movement strategies to both increase strength and functionality while minimizing pain as best as possible.

Discouragement, when it comes to movement with chronic pain, is normal. This discouragement, however, may cause patients to stop movement all together. Some patients may say, regarding their favorite physical activity or activity in general, "if I can't do it the same way, I might as well not do it at all." This statement is very dangerous. Such individuals may begin to fear the activities they previously loved. The decreased interest and discouragement to be active, as a result of chronic pain, may lead to reduced mobility overall. If this reduced mobility becomes a habit, many patients may notice it takes more effort to do the activities that were previously easier to complete. In addition, decreased mobility may lead to weight gain, systemic disease and eventually more pain.

It must be noted, however, that when you are active with chronic pain, you may not be able to be mobile as before and this is often to be expected. Do not feel like you have to move with the same physicality as your family and friends. As you learn to move with the chronic pain, pacing yourself in your fitness goals is essential. This comes with establishing short term and long-term goals about your movement, energy level, and ability to perform certain tasks.

Remember that success comes gradually with frequent training. There is great value in building your strength, rather than letting your functionality deteriorate under the stress of chronic pain.

Work and Disability

Chronic pain can have significant implications in the workplace. It has been associated with reduced performance while at work in one study by Kosuke Kawai and colleagues; chronic pain sufferers reported losing 2 hours of productivity due to their pain as compared to those without pain [2]. Such losses in performance can result in increased risk for unemployment, decreased job satisfaction, increased stress, reduced fulfillment and hindered career growth. Additionally, one may feel that she or he is unable to participate in certain types of jobs due to the physical demands associated with that line of work. The type of work required for a particular job may even directly contribute to or worsen one's existing chronic pain. If one is performing difficult manual labor for large portions of time during the week, it can result in wear and tear upon the body over time and may increase the risk of an acute injury.

Interestingly, some studies seem to indicate that the type of job one has may not be as influential to the development of chronic pain, as one might assume. Robert Teasell and Claire Bombardier performed a thorough review of the literature to try and ascertain what work characteristics may be more likely to be present for those suffering from chronic pain as compared to those whom do not. According to their efforts, it seemed that there was limited evidence suggested that physical demands of a job influence the development of chronic pain disability. Again, this may speak to the resilience of those with chronic pain. Also, of note, it appears that having a job that offers one some autonomy and flexibility to modify work activities may reduce the likelihood that someone may develop chronic pain disability [7]. Searching for job opportunities that may offer this flexibility may yield long term benefits to those at risk for developing chronic pain.

The economic cost of chronic pain upon our society is on the scale of billions of dollars a year in the United States; and such costs manifest themselves through loss of productivity while an employee is at work, loss of productivity when the employee takes time off from work and the direct medical costs supplied to cover medical and other treatments for chronic pain. Based on data from 2002, Collins and colleagues studied the financial impact chronic pain can have upon employers by examining the costs the Dow Chemical company incurred for an employee with chronic illnesses, such as back and neck disorders. Not only did they identify that chronic back and neck disorders were associated with increased work impairment and absences, but they also estimated that on average such conditions cost the firm about $10,000 dollars per employee per year, about two thirds of the costs coming from impaired working performance [8]. Such costs are most certainly higher now.

Of note, the role of compensation in the form of disability payments may play a role in how well one with chronic pain clinically improves. It has been shown that those with a financial benefit associated with their pain disability, such as work compensation, may have less improvement in their pain disability over the course of a year of rehabilitation as compared to those with compensation associated with their disability. One should be conscious of this association to prevent unnecessary stunted improvements due to other incentives. This finding may suggest that opposing motivational factors (e.g. financial benefit vs. physical improvement) may hinder rehabilitation progress for chronic pain. Also, it is possible that having a financial stake in one's chronic pain disability may result in one "buying" into the sick role and thereby making a person with chronic pain think and feel less capable of participating whole heartedly in their rehabilitation efforts. Along these lines, one should also be aware of the Family and Medical Leave Act (FMLA) in the United States, which allows for one to acquire up to 12 weeks of unpaid occupational leave due to a significant incapacitating medical condition. Some types of pain can qualify for various amounts of leave time under FMLA. It is critical to understand that each individual's situation must be assessed by a medical professional and be approved through the appropriate medical and legal channels to qualify. The purpose of this law is to preserve one's employment position, while allowing him or her the appropriate time away from work to pursue medical management and rehabilitation for their incapacitating medical issue, such as an exacerbation of chronic pain.

Sleep

Obtaining adequate quality sleep has significant implications on mental health, emotional stability, and physical wellness. It is important to recognize that chronic pain and sleep are intricately intertwined. Several studies have indicated that difficulty sleeping occurs in the majority of those with chronic pain. For example, it has been found that 53% to 90% of chronic pain patients suffer from significant insomnia. Additionally, it is believed that the severity of pain is believed to be correlated with the severity of sleep difficulty. Furthermore, sleep deprivation has been found to increase pain intensity and vice versa, thereby creating a vicious cycle of worsening sleep and worsening pain [3]. Due to the interconnected nature of sleep and chronic pain, it is important to assess the quality and quantity of sleep one is obtaining. Drug treatments for sleep disturbances may be problematic due to accompanying side effects, at times their questionable effectiveness and safety concerns [9]. Obtaining adequate sleep duration (at least 7-8 hours of quality uninterrupted sleep) can be a useful way to reduce one's chronic pain. In order to do this, improving sleep hygiene can be a great place to start. By changing sleep habits and attitude toward sleep, those suffering from chronic pain may be able to focus more on obtaining the rest the body needs in order to function properly throughout the day.

Not only does how one's sleep affect one's quality of rest, but the behaviors and environment of a patient can greatly affect their sleep and therefore the severity of the chronic pain (discussed in another chapter).

Social Life

Those with chronic pain may be concerned with their ability to function in social contexts, which may restrict their opportunities for socialization. Von Korff and colleagues found that almost 1 in 5 individuals with chronic spinal pain felt that they were unable to participate in some major social role as compared to those without chronic spinal pain [10]. Of note, chronic pain can be episodic with periods of worsening symptoms, during which, one's ability to participate in social activities may be restricted. For those that experience intermittent episodes of worsened pain, it may be gratifying to recognize that the exacerbations will end, and this idea can offer some solace. Limitations upon one's ability to partake in social activities can result in increased stress, reduced social support, altered sense of identity, and a sense of detachment. All of these effects can impact one's mood and emotional stability. As a result, pushing oneself to maintain healthy social interactions and activity is important.

It can be particularly difficult for children with chronic pain to live with the same enthusiasm or ability to operate actively in social situations as they may have done previously. Because so much of a child's time is spent in school, how academic achievement is affected by chronic pain is an important consideration. Concerning academic achievement, it can be expected that children and adolescents with chronic pain may have more school absences than their classmates. As a result of the anxiety created by the pressure of constant movement in the school environment and the distraction that chronic pain causes, it is possible that children with chronic pain may have lower academic achievement in comparison to their classmates. This same anxiety can limit a child's social interactions and ability to formulate friendships, especially since social interactions at school and during after school activities often center around activities that could exacerbate the child's pain, such as sports, recess or gym activities. Participating in other after school activities, such as singing in a choir, participating in an art class, or learning how to play an instrument, may be great ways for the child to become active in their communities and establish friendships while minimizing the anxiety associated with their chronic pain. Often, because of the lack of support within their school environment, children may heavily rely on parental figures to express their physical and emotional concerns. Discouragement resulting from not being able to complete daily activities independently or not being as active as their friends and classmates may cause a sense of hopelessness and social disconnection. It is important then, as parents, to be attentive to the behaviors of the child and ask about their feelings regarding their academic achievement, their ability to make friends, interests they are developing, as well as their level and management of pain.

Adults have many social spheres in their lives in which chronic pain can limit interaction and participation. In the family environment, the patient may feel discouraged to participate within family functions and not want their loved ones to see them suffering. Within the work environment as well as within the intimate family setting, sufferers of chronic pain may feel ashamed of their pain and their inability to contribute the same energy to a project or task as their coworkers or family members. It is important to note that within any setting, one's effortful interactions with others are valued and should therefore be encouraged. Being able to spend time with others and offer some contribution to one's community demonstrates great participatory behavior and can strengthen one's sense of determination to continue being an important player in one's various social spheres. It is very important to seek help from a specialized pain psychologist or psychiatrist if necessary

Family

There is another group of people who indirectly suffer from chronic pain: the family and loved ones of those with chronic pain. These individuals are often underappreciated, and one might call them "hidden sufferers." The status and well-being of relationships can be tested by chronic pain and may result in far reaching and significant challenges. The negative impact chronic pain has upon the family's wellness is often perceived as worse from the perspective of family members as compared to the person with the chronic pain. This is important to understand, as one with chronic pain may not fully appreciate the effect their disability and suffering can have upon their support system. It can be a draining experience for both the sufferer and the support system, so appreciating the scope and value of these partnerships can be useful. Also, demonstrating gratefulness for this support can be rewarding for both parties.

Chronic pain may become a source of tension in relationships. Some people suffering from chronic pain feel guilty for requiring assistance from family or loved ones and can feel that they are a burden upon those they love. Family members can feel limited in their ability to enjoy some activities with their loved one and can feel trapped due to the limitations their loved one's condition can place upon their lives. Either the sufferer or support giver can even lash out due to frustration with their respective situation. Additionally, it can be difficult to look on as someone you love and care about is suffering.

Through a concerned nature, the sufferer may grow to realize even further the amount of respect and sense of dignity a significant other carries for them as well as appreciate more deeply his or her nurturing abilities. In addition, living with chronic pain and the stressors it presents may overshadow other relationship challenges or alter one's perspective on their relative importance. Of course, every relationship is different, and the amount, quality, and longevity of support given to the chronic pain sufferer may differ from relationship to relationship.

The development of chronic pain may take an unexpected toll on the plans of a couple or family. The stresses and hardships associated with chronic pain can often be transferred to one's spouse or partner. In addition to the general stresses mentioned above, there are additional challenges that may arise due to disability. Being disabled may change the financial status of the household, potentially causing one partner to change his or her career trajectory or workload in order to accommodate household and personal finances. This stress may also take time away from supporting the sufferer of chronic pain, as well as participating in family or social engagements. Additionally, the need to support a family member with chronic pain may detract from time spent at work or fulfilling other responsibilities.

Being a parent becomes increasingly difficult with the stress of chronic pain, both for the sufferer and the supporter within the spousal relationship. Depending upon the disability associated with the chronic pain, the family members without chronic pain may have to assume increased levels of responsibility within the house. Such responsibilities can include more household chores, driving the children to and from school and activities, taking care of their work responsibilities, and worrying about the chronic pain of one's loved one. With the continuous pressure to complete task after task, the supporter may feel the value drain out of the activities he or she once loved.

On the other hand, the spouse with chronic pain may feel guilty for not being able to contribute to or participate in as many family activities as they would like. This is one way in which chronic pain can be not only physically strenuous, but emotionally difficult as well.

Fully appreciating the influence of chronic pain on one's children can be challenging and variable. Some research has indicated that children can express frustration with missing out on activities due to parental chronic pain, reduced communication strategies, worsened emotional stress and sadness, and increased independence earlier in childhood. Of note, some positive findings were found in some offspring, such as increased levels of compassion and empathy [11]. Logically speaking, a sufferer of chronic pain may feel jealousy towards other parent's ability to participate in activities with their children. This can be accompanied also by a feeling of guilt. Additionally, as a parent, you want to be able to stand strong by your child's side, as a protector and role model, during school functions. However, chronic pain can bring a feeling of hopelessness and weakness that may make the parent feel unfit or ashamed to be present at such functions. Overall, it once again is critical to remember that each individual is different and therefore generalizations must not be taken out of reasonable context.

Living with chronic pain can be emotionally difficult. Feelings such as fear about the future and guilt about not being able to participate in activities or contribute in ways one previously did, may arise. According to Julie Silver, a sufferer of chronic pain and his or her family may go through the Kübler-Ross 5 stages of grief. More specifically Silver indicates that chronic pain sufferers and support givers may first experience "denial" of the pain, followed by a stage of "anger" and frustration regarding the pain and its consequences. The third stage, "bargaining", signifies a point where the sufferer may begin to make internal and external deals, such as appealing to a higher power to improve his or her symptoms in exchange for a change in his or her behavior. The fourth stage of "depression" is associated with sadness and potentially feelings of detachment or loneliness. The fifth and final stage of this process is "acceptance", in which the sufferer and her or his family members come to regard pain as a part of their lives and may change their goals in terms of pain management expectations with a focus on optimizing quality of life and function. It is important to note that progression through the various stages of grief may not occur in the specific aforementioned order, and many find themselves cycling through steps multiple times or in a different order.

Through this emotional roller coaster, a support system is vital. The family or caregivers and the sufferer can find solace in one another during this time by effectively communicating the pressures and stresses felt and possibly creating a plan to spend time together doing activities they both enjoy. It may be important for a stressed caregiver to turn to extended family and friends for support. It is possible that they may offer their assistance to pick up some tasks to lighten the load. However, it is important to understand throughout this whole process, the sufferer of chronic pain may feel insecure about his or her disabilities and dependence on others. This insecurity may lead the chronic pain sufferer to feel uncomfortable asking for others' assistance. Going through chronic pain in a supportive environment is obviously beneficial. However, some individuals may find themselves in situations in which family or a support system are not readily available. This can make tackling the above-mentioned issues associated with chronic pain even more challenging. It is imperative that such individuals reach out to other resources including, support groups, health care providers and community systems or religious organizations who may be potential sources of support.

Summary

In this chapter we have briefly discussed how chronic pain can influence a number of different aspects of one's life and also how such aspects can impact one's ability to manage his or her chronic pain. This interconnectedness is appreciable and can have possible therapeutic implications. Overall, it is best to view the role chronic pain can have upon an individual within the context of their environment and lifestyle. In addition, an element of a certain environment has the capability to influence elements of another environment. For example, stress in at home can influence one's ability to perform at work, manage other life stressors, sleep, exercise, maintain other social relationships, etc. Each of the aforementioned factors can in turn influence how one feels and manages his or her chronic pain. While such an interconnected web can seem complex, it also offers many avenues for one to seek self-improvement. By selecting one element to improve upon, one may be able to reap benefits in many other areas, including improved chronic pain management! For example, improving one's sleep quality may promote more effective pain management, as well as unlock other benefits such as enhanced relationships, increased work performance, etc. Additionally, understanding the extent with which chronic pain can influence the life of the chronic pain sufferer and his or her supporters, can help one appreciate the significance of attempting self-improvement efforts. Hopefully, such efforts can snowball to further effect positive changes.

References

1. Dahlhamer J. Prevalence of Chronic Pain and High-Impact Chronic Pain Among Adults — United States, 2016. MMWR Morb Mortal Wkly Rep 2018; 67:1001-1006. https://www.cdc.gov/mmwr/volumes/67/wr/mm6736a2.htm

2. Kawai K, et al. Adverse impacts of chronic pain on health-related quality of life, work productivity, depression and anxiety in a community-based study. Fam Pract 2017; 34:656–61.

3. Dueñas M, et al. A review of chronic pain impact on patients, their social environment and the health care system. J of Pain Res 2016; 9:457–467.

4. Berg-Emons R et al. Impact of chronic pain on everyday physical activity. Euro J of Pain 2007; 11:587–93.

5. Arnstein P, et al. Self-efficacy as a mediator of the relationship between pain intensity, disability and depression in chronic pain patients. Pain 1999; 80:483–491.

6. Turk D, et al. The Pain Survival Guide: How to Reclaim Your Life. 1st ed. American Psychological Association, Washington 2006.

7. Teasell R, et al. Employment-Related Factors in Chronic Pain and Chronic Pain Disability. Clin J Pain 2001; 17: S39-S45.

8. Collins J, et al. The Assessment of Chronic Health Conditions on Work Performance, Absence, and Total Economic Impact for Employers. J Occup Environ Med 2005; 47:547-557.

9. Nijs J, et al. Sleep Disturbances in Chronic Pain: Neurobiology, Assessment, and Treatment in Physical Therapist Practice.

10. Physical Therapy 2018; 98: 325-326

11. Pitcher M, et al. Prevalence and Profile of High-Impact Chronic Pain in the United States. J Pain 2018; epub ahead of print.

12. Higgins K, et al. Offspring of Parents with Chronic Pain: A Systematic Review and Meta-Analysis of Pain, Health, Psychological, and Family Outcomes. Pain 2015; 156:2256–2266.

SUPPORTING YOUR SPOUSE

IN CHRONIC PAIN

Introduction

Pain is a complex physiological response to a host of toxic or noxious stimuli. In the acute phase, pain is an appropriate response necessary to alert us of tissue injury. However, this pain can persist, sometimes even after the acute insult is resolved. If this pain lasts longer than 12 weeks, it is aptly named chronic pain and represents a primary process itself [1]. In addition to causing physical distress, chronic pain causes significant suffering as it can carry detrimental effects to mental well-being and even produce or worsen numerous other symptoms.

Chronic pain is widely prevalent in our society; latest CDC data estimated that 50 million persons (20.4% of U.S. adults) suffer from chronic pain and that 19.6 millions of these persons (8.0% of U.S. adults) suffer from severe chronic pain [1]. Of those affected, women, elder persons, and those in lower socioeconomic strata are disproportionately affected. Due to its significant prevalence, chronic pain is one of the largest public health concerns affecting our country.

Chronic pain is a debilitating disease as it commonly affects numerous facets of daily life, such as but not limited to activities of daily living and ambulation [1,2]. Thus, many patients may even find employment or general participation in community activities to be too taxing to endure. As debilitating as a disease, chronic pain may be for patients, it can also have a profound impact on their entire families. In particular, spouses may be especially affected as they are often tasked with not only fulfilling caregiver roles, but also with assuming many of the patients' former responsibilities [2,3]. These obligations may span financial, housekeeping, and familial duties and can often provoke psychological distress in spouses [2-4]. In severe cases, this distress can propagate strife within the spousal relationship.

Due to the complex biopsychosocial determinants affecting chronic pain, affected patients can have drastically varying outcomes and levels of suffering depending on a host of external factors [2,4,5]. Spousal support is often one of the most influential factors involved in the overall health of persons with chronic pain. Therefore, strong and successful support from a spouse can reduce stressor burden for patients and promote healing and wellness [2,5].

Likewise, suboptimal support can have detrimental effects on patients' mental well-being and even hamper the recovery phase of chronic pain. Consequently, a thorough understanding of the numerous external factors affecting patients with chronic pain and the role spouses may play in this paradigm is instrumental in supporting a loved one affected by chronic pain.

Understanding Chronic Pain

The precise pathophysiology of chronic pain has yet to be clearly elucidated. Thus, managing and treating chronic pain is often challenging from a clinical standpoint. Likewise, this lack of understanding of chronic pain can also be challenging for affected persons. Even as persons with chronic pain learn to appreciate the subtleties of their disease process, a clear appreciation of the underlying etiologies may be overlooked as there exist numerous biopsychosocial factors that may be contributing to their illness [1,2,5]. Notably, major depression and other depressive disorders are known to be heavily involved in the development of chronic pain [4,5]. However, these psychological disorders require a high amount of personal insight in order to appreciate.

Just as understanding chronic pain is difficult for patients to appreciate, it can often be more challenging for their partners, especially as most chronic pain conditions are not visibly appreciable [2]. These challenges in understanding, however, should be addressed before the affected persons' spouses can become effective caregivers. By listening to their affected spouses, accompanying them to doctor's appointments, and even doing their own independent research involving the topic, unaffected spouses can begin to appreciate chronic pain and how it affects their partners.

Of note, however, unaffected spouses may be at an advantage in that they may be able to appreciate how any psychological impairments that exist affects their significant others' chronic pain [2,4,5]. In conjunction with these impairments, they may also be able to appreciate the vulnerability and hopelessness that many affected persons face early in the diagnosis. While witnessing and appreciating their partner in distress is crucial, their response as caregivers can be vital to facilitate a healthy progression through the chronic pain disease course.

Effective Interspousal Communication

Once caregiver spouses begin to understand chronic pain as a disease process, they may begin to appreciate the subtleties it entails in day to day life. Chronic pain is not a static process, but rather a dynamic impairment with episodic breakthrough pain [2,5]. This paradigm of pain often translates to waxing and waning caregiver requirements. However, affected persons may not always receive the help and support they require from these acute perturbations in pain status due to numerous reasons including pride and guilt in requesting assistance. This pattern of behavior may be maladaptive as it excludes their partners from offering their services as caregivers [2]. In order for the unaffected spouse to become an effective provider, it is the responsibility of the affected spouse to openly disclose their symptoms to their partner to facilitate open communication and allow the caregiver spouse to become more attuned to triggering stimuli and their effects.

Open communication from the caregiver spouses to their partners is also essential for a functional relationship dynamic [2,5]. If caregiver responsibilities accrue and worsen, the affected person may not always be able to predict how these new stressors can affect their caregiver spouses, especially if they are also burdened with other duties. Unaddressed, added responsibilities and requirements can produce caregiver fatigue, which can facilitate interspousal strife and disrupt effective care delivery to the affected person [2,4,5]. To prevent these dilemmas, caregiver spouses should openly communicate when responsibility become overwhelming, following which alternative strategies for caregiving can be developed.

Both the caregiver and affected spouse have much to share in this relationship dynamic. A lack of effective communication can lead to ineffective caregiving and serve to impact both parties negatively [2,3]. While open communication can prove challenging to some couples, they should understand that healthy communication can be remarkably helpful as both members progress through chronic pain and through the recovery phase.

Supporting your Spouse

After understanding the complex nature of chronic pain and more importantly how it affects their spouse, caregiver spouses are faced with numerous expectations for providing emotional and physical support [2,3]. Though this can be perceived as daunting, effective spousal support can help with chronic pain management, which then in turn may decrease caregiver requirements. However, a healthy appreciation for chronic pain pathophysiology must exist from caregiver spouses, especially early in the course of chronic pain recovery. In the early course, affected spouses can be afflicted with significant emotional and psychological vulnerability as they develop their own understanding about their disease [4,5]. Thus, in this stage of vulnerability and across the remainder of their affliction, strong and effective spousal support can be instrumental in helping manage psychological distress and ensure mental well- being, which collectively can promote the healthy biopsychosocial structure needed for chronic pain recovery.

Once affected by chronic pain, many persons are often unable to maintain their numerous pre- morbid commitments [1,2]. Even if they attempt to maintain these obligations, patients with chronic pain are often unable to fulfill these roles to their entire extents. Common roles and obligations that patients often find challenging to maintain include employment, schooling, parenting, caregiving to other family members, housekeeping, and various other community obligations. Consequently, these patients may require modifications or reductions to these roles. However, it must be noted that while some commitments, like schooling, can be readily reduced or discontinued, other perhaps more essential commitments, like housekeeping and parenting, often require caregiver support in order to fulfill. Additionally, caregivers may also be faced with financial strains in the setting of an unwell spouse being unable to fulfill full-time employment [1,2]. Therefore, it is crucial to establish if, how, and which prior obligations require modifications or caregiver support from the well spouse. Establishing healthy and reasonable parameters for spousal support can ensure healthy caregiver dynamics and prevent caregiver burden.

Addressing Caregiver Burden

The health and well-being of spouses who assume the role of caregivers are sometimes overlooked or forgotten [1-3]. Not only can caring and supporting for their loved ones be a mentally and physically taxing responsibility, but also the caregiver spouses are now void of the emotional support to which they were once accustomed. The new relationship dynamics where the caregiver spouse and the unwell spouse provide and require, respectively, physical and emotional support can prove challenging. These challenges may especially be pronounced if the concept and threat of caregiver burden is not readily acknowledged.

It is a known phenomenon that the risk of psychological distress, and even depressive disorders, affecting caregivers is linearly correlated with the intensity and duration of support that they provide for their unwell spouses [2,3]. Moreover, once developed, these depressive disorders can be challenging to treat and manage, especially if the caregiver support stressors continue to persist. Treating and managing depression is often difficult as, like most mental illnesses, it is not visibly appreciated. Even if diagnosed appropriately, effective treatment can be challenging. Therefore, preventing caregiver burden altogether is ultimately the most effective approach in ensuring caregiver mental wellness.

In the context of a spouse of chronic pain, it is also known that their mental and physical well- being is heavily dependent on that of their caregiver spouses. Simply put, suboptimal support provided by caregivers can be detrimental to chronic pain recovery [2,3,5]. This suboptimal support can be delivered when the caregiver is burdened by psychological stressors, as previously discussed, or even physical impairments. Regardless of the cause, persons with chronic pain can develop mental distress and their own psychological impairments when tasked with providing for themselves to a greater degree.

Interestingly, and rather unfortunately, mental distress and overt psychological disorders are known to worsen numerous chronic pain conditions [2,4,5]. Worsened chronic pain can subsequently then increase caregiver requirements, which if and when unmet can further worsen and propagate this vicious cycle. Therefore, if overwhelmed by the immensity of caregiver needs required, it is prudent for caregiver spouses to recruit assistance in order to ensure that their unwell spouses can receive the appropriate care.

Social Support

As briefly discussed in prior sections, chronic pain has the potential to affect entire families of affected persons [2]. While spouses can often fulfill caregiver roles, they may be susceptible to caregiver burden if the unwell spouse requires a large amount of support [3]. Especially in cases where affected persons had multiple pre-morbid roles and duties, the degree of caregiver support can often be overwhelming. The caregiver spouse may, unfortunately, be unable to fulfill all their unwell spouse's roles in addition to maintaining their own roles and any new roles that arise with the debility of chronic pain. Sometimes, this amount of support, either mental or physical, can be significant enough to require multiple caregivers. Regardless the specific paradigm, a healthy social support system can help compensate for overwhelming caregiver requirements and even provide persons with chronic pain with emotional reassurance from multiple persons [2,3,5].

While social support can be useful to alleviate physical caregiver requirements, it can also be instrumental in providing the emotional support that many patients with chronic pain lack [2- 5]. Even if they receive a healthy and appropriate amount of emotional support from their caregiver spouses, patients with chronic pain can be reaffirmed with positive social support. This assurance can even help alleviate any mental anguish or distress patients experience about their chronic pain illness. Therefore, implementing effective social support structures is encouraged to mitigate mental distress and possibly even prevent chronic pain exacerbation.

Sexual Dysfunction

Just as chronic pain is impacted by a plethora of biopsychosocial factors, so too is sexual well- being [2]. In the case of chronic pain, afflicted persons often possess several physical impairments related to their chronic pain diagnosis. These primary disease states, which can range from cancer to spinal surgery, pose various physical barriers to sexual health. In regard to chronic pain, disease states like pelvic pain can also present physical barriers that preclude sexual intercourse. Irrespective of these physical impairments, there also exist many psychological barriers that can prevent mutually enjoyable sexual intercourse. Unfortunately, many couples, where one member is suffering from chronic pain, often report a reduction in sexual activity, unenjoyable intercourse, or even complete sexual aversion.

Depression is thought to be one of the most prevailing causes of sexual dysfunction in persons suffering from chronic pain [2,4,5]. It is thought to precipitate a decrease in libido and sexual interest, which may lead to a lack of emotional and physical intimacy. Therefore, appropriate management of depression may be necessary to ensure that healthy sexual intercourse can proceed. It should also be noted that caregiver spouses may also have mental barriers that preclude them from participating in sexual activity with their unwell spouses. Notably, caregivers may develop what are sometimes unhealthy attitudes about physical intimacy with their sick partners. Managing these attitudes through a healthy understanding of their spouse's current disease state can be useful. Lastly, strife within the relationship can also be a common etiology of sexual dysfunction, and it is one that arises from both persons in the relationship [2- 5]. Strife can develop from overburdened caregivers who may develop animosity towards their unwell spouses and, likewise, from affected partners who believe they may not be receiving the adequate amount of support from their caregiver spouses. Reestablishing healthy parameters for spousal expectations and caregiver support can help alleviate strife and promote the emotional wellness necessary for a healthy sexual relationship.

Financial Strain

Due to the host of physical impairments and restrictions associated with their chronic pain diagnosis, affected patients are often unable to continue their full-time employment commitments [1,2]. Rather, patients often require part time employment or even leaves of absence in order to ensure that available time is more appropriately spent with more essential duties like parenting or housekeeping. With this reduction in employment and subsequent monetary income, financial strain often becomes a source of contention for several affected couples

[2,6]. This problem gets further compounded by ongoing healthcare expenses that may be accompanying the chronic pain disease process. It is noteworthy that healthcare expenses are a common cause of debt and bankruptcy in the United States. Therefore, establishing a rational fiscal plan for compensating for diminished household income in the context of ongoing healthcare expenses is necessary to prevent or reduce financial strain [6]. If unaddressed, the degree of financial strain may grow and be associated with a congruent degree of strife within the relationship [4-6].

While chronic pain poses numerous psychological and physical challenges, as aforementioned, financial responsibility is also an important factor that warrants early recognition and response. Also aforementioned are the challenges caregiver spouses can face is continuing their own employment in a full-time capacity while caring for their unwell partners. By understanding and organizing all the caregiver support required by the affected person, couples can appropriately distribute the required support across their social support structures such that they can optimize the caregiver spouse's time and efforts [2,3,5,6]. With this appropriation of tasks and support requirements, couples may find that the well spouse's efforts may be best spent maintaining their full-time employment to ensure a steady household income, while other parties help deliver the needed care for caregiving. Similarly, other couples may find that they prefer the well spouse to assume the role of a primary caregiver and sacrifice full time employment. While this strategy may be appropriate for some, these couples should also have a plan in place to address their ongoing financial requirements.

Seek help

Both the patient and the spouse/caregiver should seek help whenever they think they cannot handle the burdens of chronic pain in all aspects discussed above. Consulting with a psychiatrist or a psychologist might be necessary to address the psychological burdens in the relationship.

Marriage counseling, seeking financial aid, caregiving aid and social support might help alleviate the burden on both the patient and the spouse.

Summary

Chronic pain is a devastating illness that affects the entire family. Unfortunately, the precise mechanisms underlying chronic pain have yet to be clearly delineated. This lack of clear understanding makes dealing with this illness challenging to affected persons. Similarly, spouses of persons with chronic pain are faced with numerous challenges from understanding the implicated disease process to effectively provide the necessary emotional and physical support. Additionally, caregiver spouses are also tasked with navigating around numerous barriers to providing this support including caregiver burden and financial strains. While challenging, by maintaining a channel of open communication with their affected spouses, caregiver spouses can ameliorate some of the mental and physical stressors that challenge affected patients. By diminishing these stressors, wellness and recovery of chronic pain can be facilitated.

One of the main challenges facing couples where a member is affected by chronic pain is the prospect that new relationship dynamics are necessary to be established. The goal of progressing through the chronic pain disease time course is not to expect and attain a normal pre-morbid relationship; these expectations may be unreasonable. Rather, understanding that this affliction presents a formidable challenge to both parties and warrants new relationship dynamics. This new relationship – one of an unwell partner who requires the support of a caregiver spouse – is necessary to successfully traverse chronic pain through the disease phase and to the recovery stages. It is important for the patient and the spouse to seek all kinds of help to ensure their relationship well-being.

References

1. Dahlhamer, J, et al. Prevalence of chronic pain and high-impact chronic pain among adults—United States, 2016. Morbidity and Mortality Weekly Report, 2018; 67(36), p.1001.

2. Roy, R. Chronic pain and family: A clinical perspective. Springer Science & Business Media, 2006.

3. Adelman, R.D et al. Caregiver burden: a clinical review. Jama, 2014; 311(10), p.1052-1060.

4. Clark, M.R. et al. Pain and depression: an interdisciplinary patient-centered approach (Vol. 25). Karger Medical and Scientific Publishers, 2006.

5. Moore, R.J. Biobehavioral approaches to pain. New York, NY: Springer 2009.

6. Skinner, M.A., Zautra, A.J. and Reich, J.W. Financial stress predictors and the emotional and physical health of chronic pain patients. Cognitive Therapy and Research, 2004; 28(5), p.695-713.

SUPPORTING YOUR PARENTS

IN CHRONIC PAIN

Introduction

The population is aging in the United States, and aging presents a number of challenges. Not least among these is chronic pain, which is a common occurrence for elderly individuals. In fact, one national study concluded that greater than 50% of adults age 65 or older experienced bothersome pain sometime in the past month [1].

Chronic pain impacts patients as well as their families, with ramifications including loss of appetite, impaired sleep, physical disability, mood disorders such as depression, and cognitive decline. Taken in sum, this leads to sizable decreases in the quality of life of elderly persons with chronic pain.

This chapter will review characteristics of pain in elderly patients, as well as the impact to their lives and to the lives of their loved ones.

Elderly persons are at elevated risk for pain

As mentioned above, one national study concluded that greater than 50% of elderly individuals experienced bothersome pain in the past month [1]. This corresponds to nearly 19 million individuals in the United States, a figure greater than the combined populations of New York, Los Angeles, Chicago, and Houston. It can affect all individuals regardless of gender, race, or life history.

Pain is a common symptom of many disease processes that are associated with aging. For example, osteoarthritis causes pain in the joints, and becomes more common with advancing age. Back pain is a particularly common source of chronic pain for all Americans; however elderly individuals are at particularly high risk. Other painful conditions that are associated with the aging process include osteoporosis, diabetes, and cancer, among others.

Pain affects both the body and the mind

Functional status is a way of measuring a person's ability to perform the many activities that are required to meet the basic needs of living independently. This includes physical tasks such as the ability to bathe, dress, and purchase groceries, but can also be limited by cognitive issues such as depression or dementia. Pain can significantly decrease an individual's functional status as they age. Everyday tasks that were once simple, such as preparing meals, cleaning, or walking to the mailbox, can become insurmountably difficult in the face of chronic pain. In addition, pain can rob elderly individuals of their balance and coordination; this can lead to falls or other injuries that both create more pain and require expensive medical intervention, leading to a cycle of worsening pain and declining functional status.

Pain is a complex emotional experience that goes well beyond, for example, inadvertently touching a hot stovetop. While, in the past, much research has focused on the molecular mechanisms of pain (e.g. the specific nerve routes that pain signals traverse on their way to the brain) a comprehensive approach has more recently emerged. The biopsychosocial model views a person's pain experience as including dynamic interactions between the body, mind, and society. The interplay between these relationships provide an explanation for how a person's state of mind can influence their pain experience, and vice versa. For example, emotions such as anger or hopelessness have been shown to intensify the experience of painful stimuli [2]. And the old saying – that "laughter is the best medicine" – can be framed within the context of the biopsychosocial model to explain why a positive mood can diminish a person's pain experience. Similarly, pain can prevent individuals from engaging in social or recreational activities and thereby create a sense of isolation which, in turn, can worsen the experience of pain itself. This effect can be compounded by other negative psychological consequences of aging such as bereaving the deaths of spouses, friends and other loved ones. This method of thinking can also help explain the close relationship between chronic pain and mood disorders such as depression or anxiety in elderly individuals.

Diagnosing pain can be difficult in elderly patients

Patient self-report is considered the gold standard for diagnosis of pain. Although blood work, laboratory evaluation, or imaging studies can clue physicians in as to what a patient is likely to be experiencing, every individual ultimately experiences pain in his or her own way.

Healthcare providers will commonly measure pain severity with one of several scales to track changes in pain states and help determine the effectiveness of treatments. Although there are many, one of the most commonly used is the Numeric Rating Scale (i.e. "On a scale from 0 to 10 (10 being the worst), how bad is your pain today?"). In elderly persons who have coexisting cognitive decline, pain scales such as the Numeric Rating Scale may be difficult to understand. There are other pain measurement tools that can be used in this circumstance, such as the Faces Scale (where patients select from a number of facial expressions communicating escalating levels of discomfort) or the Pain Thermometer (asking patients to mark along a continuous scale to convey their pain severity from cool to hot). Even these scales require some level of cooperation on the part of the patient, however, which can be difficult in cases of dementia or severe depression. Specific nonverbal cues such as groaning, slouching or other postural changes, or behavioral changes such as withdrawal can also provide valuable information to indicate an underlying pain state. In addition to these scales and signs, obtaining feedback from loved ones and/or caregivers is critical to reliably gauge the severity of a patient's pain.

Some evidence suggests that pain thresholds may be higher in elderly patients, however this conclusion certainly does not apply to all individuals [3]. Some elderly people will deny being in pain because they think that it is just a normal part of the aging process, that it is something they need to accept and live with stoically. Others might deny pain due to fear of losing their independence or becoming a burden to loved ones who wish to care for them.

Whatever the barriers, it is important to identify and understand pain in elderly individuals because this is the first step toward treatment.

Treating pain requires a multifaceted approach

As part of a comprehensive pain assessment, a physician will ask questions about the characteristics of a patient's pain and how it impacts their life, as well as perform an assessment of the patient's mood, cognitive status, and ability to perform activities of daily living such as dressing, eating, and various household duties. Beyond this, it is important to also assess a patient's support structure and access to resources within their community. This information is critical to inform the specific treatment plans for a given patient. A comprehensive treatment plan for chronic pain requires communication between multiple health care providers, the patient, and the patient's loved ones, and can include medications, physical therapy, behavioral therapy, and other techniques.

Elderly patients are at increased risk for adverse effects from medications due to numerous factors including age-related decreases in lean body mass, liver and kidney function. In addition, pain medications can interact with medications used to treat other chronic conditions, causing side effects that are sometimes difficult to predict. For this reason, physicians will commonly start with small doses, and attempt to prescribe as few medications as possible with the goal to minimize side effects and maximize a patient's ability to adhere to the regimen.

Behavioral therapy can provide patients with coping strategies and other tools to manage the experience of their pain. This can range from relatively simple strategies such as deep breathing, meditation, or distraction techniques, all the way to a formal evaluation by a pain psychologist. Support groups can foster a sense of community with other individuals who are facing similar challenges. Depending on an individual's belief structure, spiritual services may also be an important subset of behavioral therapy. For example, a Chaplain may be able to affect a certain level of comfort or trust with a deeply religious individual that other medical providers are unable to achieve. Coexisting neurologic or psychiatric diseases such as dementia, depression, or anxiety are commonly associated with chronic pain in the elderly. Depending on the severity, these conditions may warrant treatment by a mental health specialist such as a psychiatrist or geriatrician.

Physical and/or occupational therapy can also be critical to help elderly patients regain or maintain the ability to perform activities of daily living and safely care for themselves. While exercises can be pursued independently, a formal evaluation by a trained physical therapist can provide a tailored plan to address strength, flexibility, balance, and coordination.

Social support structure is necessary to allow for elderly patients to adhere to any treatment plan. Even if an appropriate pain regimen is established, elderly patients are at increased risk for imperfect adherence to the treatment plan due to issues such as cognitive decline and lack of access to transportation or funding that others may take for granted.

Interventions such as multi-dose packaging – where medications are partitioned before arriving to the patient according to when they should be administered – can help improve medication safety and adherence to treatment plans, and these services are offered by many pharmacies.

Even individuals who are still competent to live independently may require assistance with managing the many medical appointments that commonly accompany the aging process. This may require help not only with setting and maintaining a complex schedule of appointments with various medical providers, but also support with comprehending medical information and marshalling community resources in order to carry out treatment plans. Accompanying patients to their appointments and requesting written documentation of visit summaries can help ensure that medical information does not become misunderstood or forgotten. And, while younger individuals may find convenience in the increasing emphasis placed on web-based resources for health care organizations (e.g. scheduling apps, online communication of test results, etc.) this can be overwhelming for older individuals who are less tech-savvy. Regardless of health, all individuals should be advised to discuss and file legal documentation such as Healthcare Power-of-Attorney (HCPOA); this provides important clarification and is useful in many circumstances even beyond end-of-life discussions. In the setting of cognitive decline or other issues precluding the safety of independent living, professional services such as home care, assisted-living facilities or nursing homes may be warranted.

Relationships with family and caregivers are also affected

Poorly controlled pain can affect an individual's relationships with friends, family, and caregivers. Health problems for aging parents affect relationships with their adult children, and chronic pain is no different.

This relationship change can be positive. For example, increased closeness can develop as part of the trajectory of caring for aging family members. Other times, however, relationships can take negative turns as feelings of anger or resentment develop from the burden assigned to the lives of adult children when worsening pain causes an elderly parent to become increasingly dependent. These negative emotions can become exacerbated when adult children experience certain stressors in their own lives such as financial instability or problems within their own nuclear families. Although relationship characteristics are highly variable across individuals, investigators have identified several best practices that can increase the likelihood that these relationship changes will be positive. These include accurate perception of pain, open communication between family members, and refinement of coping behaviors [4]:

- Pain perception: As mentioned previously, it can be difficult for others to accurately assess the presence or intensity of another person's pain. This uncertainty can lead to negative relationship changes if, for example, an adult child doesn't understand the reasons underlying an aging parent's limitations in activity or perceived withdrawal within a relationship. Conversely, if an adult child can recognize their parent's pain, then their relationship may be more supportive.

- Open communication: In addition to allowing for accurate perception of pain, open communication can provide opportunity for children to sympathize with their parent's suffering.

- Use of coping behaviors: Coping strategies allow persons suffering from pain to better manage their responses to pain, but also allow for family members and caregivers to better manage the increased stress placed on their interpersonal relationships.

Relationships are subject to additional stress when an adult child takes the responsibility of caregiver for a parent with chronic pain. Although daily interactions have the potential to increase closeness between a caregiver child and elderly parent with pain, the challenges of managing chronic pain can take a toll on the physical and mental state of the caregiver. For example, caregivers may be forced to shuffle work responsibilities or even miss work days in order to prioritize care appointments for their loved ones or to provide support with activities of daily living. These sacrifices can send reverberations through caregivers' own nuclear families if financial or other stressors mount. Even in the absence of financial hardships, it can be difficult for adult children to see their aging parents struggle on a daily basis. Especially if pain is associated with a progressive – or even incurable – disease, everyday close contact with an aging parent can result in significant emotional trauma. In addition to their aging parents, caregivers themselves can suffer from depression or other mental health issues. Examples such as these illustrate the sizeable impact that these responsibilities can make on the lives of caregivers. This realization is paramount for adult children who do not take the role of primary caregiver (due to geographic separation, time constraints, or a variety of other reasons), as it is important for these individuals to provide support not only for their aging parents but also for their caregiving family members.

Self-care is paramount

As mentioned, adult children can experience increased stress as a result of caring for a parent with chronic pain. This stress can lead to adverse physical and emotional effects and demands appropriate attention. Individuals manage stress in various ways and there is no magic solution that is universally applicable, but there are several techniques that may be considered:

- Develop awareness of your own feelings and emotions. What stressors are contributing? Once these stressors are identified, ask for help from family and/or close friends. Even if other family members are separated geographically and would be unavailable for day-to-day in-person assistance, everyone can contribute in their own way. It is rare that a single adult child must shoulder the entire burden of caregiving.

- Understand that you control how you react to stress, even if the sources of stress are beyond your control. Coping mechanisms can be physical (e.g. deep breathing or progressive muscle relaxation) as well as psychological (e.g. meditation or reframing techniques to view the causes underpinning your reactions).

- Communication is key. Communication with your parent can allow you to better understand his or her symptoms. Communication with your spouse or other loved ones can help lift feelings of stress. This may allow you to release negative thoughts and feelings in order to help you focus on the value that you provide as a caregiver.

Just as support groups exist for patients, they are also an option for adult children caregivers. The opportunity to share ideas and learn how other individuals manage their many responsibilities can provide invaluable insight. There are also resources available to help offset the burden placed on primary caregivers. Although it is not ubiquitous, some insurance companies offer coverage for respite care, a service that will provide care for a short while (i.e. hours-to-days) to allow primary caregivers time to manage other requirements in their lives. In addition, primary caregivers may be eligible for coverage through the Family and Medical Leave Act (FMLA); your physician's office can provide more information on appropriate utilization of this resource. It is also important to set boundaries and, to the best of your ability, maintain them. Caregivers must live their own lives first, and if the amount of support becomes so great as to prevent this from occurring then perhaps it would be appropriate to consider engaging professional services such as home care or even assisted-living.

Summary

- Chronic pain is common among elderly individuals from all walks of life and is associated with significant physical and cognitive decline.

- The biopsychosocial model helps to explain the complex interactions between body, mind, and society which beget a patient's pain experience.

- Diagnosing pain in elderly individuals can be challenging for a number of reasons, not least of which is increased prevalence of depression and dementia that makes communication difficult.

- Treatment regimens may include medications as well as physical and behavioral therapy techniques.

- In addition to the patients and their spouses, chronic pain in elderly persons can impact relationships with adult children and other family members. Caregivers, especially, are exposed to increased stress in these relationships.

References

1. Patel KV, et al, Turk DC. "Prevalence and Impact of Pain among Older Adults in the United States: Findings from the 2011 National Health and Aging Trends Study." Pain. 2013;154(12): 10.1016/j.pain.2013.07.029.

2. Burns JW, et al. "Anger arousal and behavioral anger regulation in everyday life among patients with chronic low back pain: Relationships to patient pain and function." Health Psychol. 2015;34(5):547-555.

3. Lautenbacher S, et al. "Age changes in pain perception: A systematic-review and meta-analysis of age effects on pain and tolerance thresholds." Neurosci Biobehav Rev. 2017; 75:104-113.

4. Riffin C, et al. "Impact of Pain on Family Members and Caregivers of Geriatric Patients." Clin Geriatr Med. 2016;32(4):663-675.

ALGORITHM FOR TREATING

CHRONIC PAIN

Introduction

Chronic pain can be very challenging to treat. Patients with chronic pain may have their first encounter for treatment with their primary care provider, spine surgeon, orthopedic surgeon, emergency room physician, neurologist, psychiatrist, or pain management doctor.

Unfortunately, providers practice pain management differently, a surgeon may suggest surgery, primary care providers may offer medications, and pain specialists may offer interventional procedures. It is very important that patients learn about their treatment options, so they can bring their own ideas to discuss with their health care providers. This will make sure their management is implemented in an algorithm that can ensure they are getting the appropriate treatment.

We will be discussing in this chapter a proposed algorithm for the management of chronic pain. We recommend patients follow this algorithm to make sure they are getting the appropriate treatment no matter which provider they see first.

Topic

One of the very popular algorithms for treating chronic pain is the World Health Organization (WHO) ladder. This ladder was developed mainly for the treatment of cancer pain, but it is a very good algorithm for treating all chronic pain conditions.

The ladder recommends starting with less invasive modalities and ends with more invasive modalities at the top.

Step 1: Non-pharmacologic therapies. These includes modalities such as physical therapy, acupuncture, healthy nutrition, massage therapy, and more (discussed in another chapter). Sometimes this is all that is needed to treat chronic pain without the need for medications or any interventions. These modalities are also essential even if the patient will be started on medications or other treatment modalities. Performing the prior non-pharmacologic therapies will improve the efficacy of the other additional modalities.

Step 2: Add non-opioids. This step includes using medications such as antidepressants, antiseizure, over-the-counter, and other medications to treat chronic pain (discussed in chapters 9 and 10). There is very good evidence on the efficacy of using non-opioid medications for treating chronic pain. In fact, several of these agents are specifically FDA approved for treating certain chronic pain conditions.

Step 3: Mild opioids.

Step 4: Strong opioids.

Step 3 and 4 are reasonable for cancer pain treatment, but when it comes to chronic pain management, the use of opioids is not recommended. Chronic use of opioids can be harmful to patients. Low dose opioids might be appropriate for some patients who fail all other modalities in treating chronic pain, but they are not for everyone. The decision to use opioids in chronic pain should be discussed with the healthcare provider. Patients should understand the risks, opioid agreements, pill counts, checking the state registry for opioid prescriptions, and random urine drug screens that are essential to ensure compliance and reduce harm (please read chapter 13 for hazards of opioids).

Step 5: Pain procedures/interventions. There are variable procedures and interventions performed by pain providers to treat chronic pain. Providers should start with less invasive procedures as steroid injections and then move to more advanced procedures if simple procedures were not effective. Details on procedures are discussed in chapters 11 and 12.

I believe this algorithm is a very effective approach and hope all providers will use it for treating chronic pain to ensure that patients will be treated the same way no matter who is treating them.

While this algorithm is very effective, sometimes it is hard to follow in a stepwise order from step 1 to 5. Sometimes the cause of pain requires surgery right away, as in case of severe disc bulge associated with motor weakness or sensory loss. Some patients may request pain procedures during their first visit as their job will prevent them from using medications that can have side effects as sedation/drowsiness or simply because they want to see quick improvement.

That is why the first visit to manage chronic pain is extremely important to make the appropriate diagnosis and to determine a plan. The WHO ladder is an effective algorithm for treating chronic pain but sometimes exceptions will be needed to be to tailor the treatment plan to the patient's situation and condition.

Summary

The WHO ladder is an effective algorithm for treating chronic pain. It ensures appropriate management of chronic pain. Exceptions may be needed to be applied depending on patient's condition and needs. Use of opioids is not recommended for chronic pain patients, but definitely needed in certain situations. A full discussion about the plan and the risks/ benefits of each therapy is essential to make sure patient is willing to take the risk of any proposed treatment.

References

1- http://www.who.int/cancer/palliative/painladder/en/

NON-PHARMOLOGICAL THERAPIES FOR TREATING CHRONIC PAIN

Introduction

Non-pharmacological therapies can be extremely effective in the multidisciplinary approach to treating chronic pain conditions. There are a variety of treatments addressing multiple body systems. People are most successful when their support system understands these non-pharmacological therapies and helps them follow the treatment plan. This may include doing exercises with the patient, taking the patient to appointments, advocating for the patient when something isn't going well and helping the patient to understand the reason why he/she needs to perform some of these therapies. This chapter will briefly discuss several modalities that can help in treating chronic pain. If patient is interested in learning more about any of these modalities, we recommend using more resources and talking to a specialist.

Physical Therapy

Physical therapy (PT) is often part of the multidisciplinary approach to pain management. PT is a function and goal-based treatment. During your initial assessment appointment your physical therapist will ask many questions about pain and symptoms, physical function, activity tolerance and daily activities. Examples of functions are walking, dressing lower part of the body, sitting, driving, lifting, carrying, bathing, going to the bathroom, among many others.

During the first visit with a physical therapist, the patient will help to set these goals. Physical therapists use SMART goals. A SMART goal is Specific, Measurable, Achievable, Realistic and Time Bound. As your treatment progresses, the patient and the physical therapist will return to these goals and adjust the treatment plan accordingly to meet these function-based goals.

Physical therapists can use many tools to help the patient with posture, joint range of motion, strength, flexibility, pain treatment and coping strategies. These treatments match the physical impairments that physical therapist found during the initial assessment appointment. While some treatments are designed to decrease immediate pain such as soft tissue work, stretching and joint mobilization (physical therapist stretches patient's joint with their hands or other tools), home exercise program is extremely important to continue to improve or keep the gains achieved in the physical therapy visit.

Strength training: When a patient is in pain there is a reflex to decrease muscular contraction in one area and increase in another area. With acute pain (sudden onset, new pain) this can be protective and serve as a splint for the injured area. In chronic pain this reflex is no longer helpful. This reflex actually starts to cause muscles to become weaker. This leads to an imbalance in the body making it less efficient. In other words, muscles have to work harder to do the same action, such as getting out of bed, climbing stairs, or going for a walk. Prolonged time of rest also can make muscles weaker. These two factors together will amplify or increase your mechanical imbalance in the body. Anatomical changes such as osteoarthritis or degenerative disc disease are aggravated by these mechanical imbalances. PT works to find these imbalances, give the correct exercises to decrease the painful splinting actions of muscles and to strengthen the weaker areas.

There are two different types of strength training: power or moving strength and endurance or stabilizing strength. The body needs both types of strength for optimal function. Oftentimes neuromuscular re-education is also required. Neuromuscular re-education of muscles and nerves means that nerves send the right message to your muscles at the right time for the right amount of muscle contraction. People who experience chronic pain often have impaired activation of their muscles due to the reflex to protect the body. Consistent strength training will correct this.

Physical therapists may prescribe exercises such as 3 sets of 8 repetitions, 3 times per week. This is a typical power or moving strength prescription. Typically, a day of rest is included as patient will be sore from the exercise the day after. This is normal and call delayed onset muscular soreness or DOMS. DOMS can be perceived as painful, but it is important to note that this pain is beneficial as it stimulates your body to build more muscular tissue.

Physical therapists may also prescribe endurance or stabilizing strength training. The typical prescription may be 4 sets of 15 repetitions, 2 times per day. This trains muscles to hold the body up against gravity for the entire day. These exercises also train muscles and nerves to work on correct timing of contraction for patient's activities, such as getting out of bed or into and out of the vehicle. This will decrease overall joint and muscle pain as less stress is applied to the body. Getting nerves to send the right messages to muscles helps the muscles to work to their best ability.

Stretching: Physical therapists may prescribe stretching exercises to assist muscles and joints to work more efficiently. When one side of a joint is tight, the other side of the joint and its muscles have to work hard to get the joint to move. Flexibility decreases naturally as a person ages. Keeping up with good flexibility is essential for muscle, joint and nerve health. Healthy muscles, joints and nerves decrease persistent pain.

Posture: This isn't just something that a parent or grandparent talked about. Optimal posture is defined as the alignment of the human body that stabilizes the joints against gravity with the least amount of muscular activation for endurance and prolonged ability to tolerate gravity.

This optimal posture is often referred to as standard posture. To get an understanding of standard posture, the patient needs to understand the alignment of the spine and other joints at rest. This is usually done by observation or using a plumb line, the line of gravity should pass through specific points of the body if it is to be called ideal posture. On examination the body should be viewed from four aspects; front, back, and sides (left and right). The ideal "normal" erect posture is one in which the line of gravity (the vertical line drawn through the body's center of gravity) can be viewed from each side runs [1]. Prolonged periods of pain cause a person to rest in the least painful posture. While this is helpful for acute pain, in chronic pain this causes muscles to become weak, joints and muscles to become stiff and less flexible, and underlying anatomical problems to become aggravated. Physical or occupational therapists will work with the patient on the underlying problems related to impaired posture with stretching, strengthening and neuromuscular re-education to improve posture. This means the body will have to expend less energy to be upright against gravity which helps with pain, fatigue, and overall tolerance to activity.

Graded exposure to exercise: Physical therapists will guide patient to increase his/her activity level at a slow rate to allow for the body to adjust. It is important when performing graded exposure to exercise that the patient consistently perform the exercise to gain maximum benefit.

Pacing of activity: Physical and occupational therapists can teach pacing strategies to help the patient achieve all his/her functional goals for the day. When the patient is experiencing persistent or chronic pain, scheduled rest breaks with pacing the activity will allow the patient to accomplish more in the day.

Joint Protection: Many people who experience persistent or chronic pain may have anatomical changes in their joints such as osteoarthritis or degenerative disc disease. Protecting joints from overuse is an important part of the pain management plan. Daily plan for joint protection decreases the risk of pain flares and joint irritation. For example, avoid twisting and awkward positions as reaching out to objects at the back seat in a car.

Ergonomic assessment and modification: Many people use computers and technology throughout their day. Ensuring the best posture is used during these activities can lead to improved pain control. Physical and occupational therapists provide these services.

Desensitization therapy and Graded Motor Imagery: These are treatment approaches used for some chronic pain conditions. It is a series of exercises designed to change how the brain interprets the body and how the body sends messages to the brain. These exercises decrease the sensitivity of tissues and improve the messaging to the brain from one of danger to a more normal message of touch, hot, cold, pressure, etc. [2]. For example, in some diseases as complex regional pain syndrome, the patient may feel severe pain to touch. There are several strategies that can help with this kind of treatment including:

- Left/right discrimination: Research shows people in pain often lose the ability to identify left or right images of their painful body part. With special training strategies this ability to discriminate between the two sides can be achieved.

- Explicit motor imagery: The patient will be thinking about moving without actually moving. Imagining movement in patients with pain can be very hard. By imagining movements, patient uses similar brain areas as you would when you actually move.

- Mirror therapy: By putting the left hand behind a mirror and right hand in front, patient can trick his/her brain into believing that the reflection of the right hand in the mirror is the left hand.

Modalities: These are tools that physical therapists use to decrease pain, improve flexibility or change the environment in which the body is functioning. Some examples of this are listed below.

Warm water aquatic therapy: use of a warm water pool typically 90-93 degrees to increase body temperature. The buoyancy of the water takes stress off joints. This allows the patient to move more freely than would on land. Heat from the water increases blood flow to areas of the body that are sore and/or tight. Oftentimes people are able to perform more exercise than on land leading to improved flexibility, posture and strength.

Cool water aquatic therapy: similar to warm water aquatic therapy as the buoyancy allows the body to move more freely. Typically, cool water is used when a person's medical conditions do not allow for the higher temperature or access to a warm water pool is unavailable.

TENS unit: transcutaneous electrical nerve stimulation (TENS) units provide an electrical current to change how the body interacts with the pain signal. There are a variety of types of nerve stimulation including continuous, modulation, burst, and a combination of these. Certain patients should not use a TENS unit. Patients should consult with their medical team to see if this may be an option.

Other treatments are available such as traction, ultrasound, laser and dry needling [3], among others. Research is mixed on the benefits of these treatments for chronic pain as the treatment effect is short lasting. Physical or occupational therapist can evaluate if these other treatments are beneficial for patient.

Occupational Therapy

Occupational therapists are similar to physical therapists in providing a variety of treatment interventions. Depending on where patient lives, physical and occupational therapists focus on different treatments. Many occupational therapists will work on energy conservation, activity planning, joint protection, stretching, strength training, and posture retraining. Additionally, they may utilize braces, or orthotics to decrease pain and improve function.

Tai Chi

Tai Chi is an ancient Chinese exercise form used for both defense and health benefits. There are different types of tai chi in addition to different levels of difficulty. Tai Chi Fundamentals® developed by David Braga, Jill Johnson, and Tricia Yu focuses on the basic moves in Tai Chi exercise to make this more accessible to persons with physical impairments or limitations. Tai chi focuses on mid-range of motion of joints, balance, breathing, strength training of the legs and trunk and has excellent functional applications. Tai Chi can be adapted to be performed in sitting with one hand support or standing.

Yoga

Yoga is a group of physical, mental and spiritual practices that originated in ancient India. In addition to the physical exercises performed in yoga, it has a meditation core.

There are different types of yoga in addition to different difficulty levels. Persons with chronic pain trying yoga should look for a beginner's class that performs poses separately so that patient can pay close attention to how the body is moving. Yoga focuses on breathing, elongating the body, stretching with strength at the end range of motion of joints, and balance. Yoga can be adapted to be performed in sitting, standing or lying down. Yoga can also be performed in different air temperatures which changes how the body will stretch, similar to aquatic therapy. Yoga has been shown to improve physical, psychological, and social health quality of life [4].

Meditation

Meditation is the practice where a person uses certain strategies such as mindfulness or focus their mind on an object, thought or activity to train attention and awareness and achieve and mentally and emotionally clear calm state. Meditation can be used to reduce stress, anxiety and pain.

Meditation has been studied in many patient populations. One recent study focused on knee osteoarthritis and chronic pain associated with this anatomical condition. The findings of this exploratory study suggested that a simple meditative mantra may be effective in reducing knee pain and dysfunction, decreasing stress, and improving mood, sleep, and quality of life in adults with knee osteoarthritis [5].

Acupuncture

Acupuncture is the placement of thin needles through the skin in certain strategic points in the body.

The traditional Chinese medicine explains acupuncture as a technique used for balancing the flow of energy-known as chi or qi (chee)-which is believed to flow through certain pathways (meridians) in the body. By inserting needles into specific points along these meridians, energy flow will re-balance.

Its therapeutic effects on pain have been validated by both basic and clinical research, and it is currently emerging as a unique non-pharmaceutical choice for pain against the opioid crisis [6,7].

Support System

A support system is extremely important for persons experiencing chronic persistent pain. Care givers can drive the patient to appointments, attend exercise group therapy or classes, and perform exercises with them at home. Holding a person with chronic pain accountable for their actions is also very important. Care givers should support healthy decisions regarding pacing of activity, graded exposure to exercise, and encourage appropriate prescribed medication use. Patients should learn about how the pain system works so they may empathize without pity. Care givers can also assist patients with scheduling regular visits or exercise time. In addition, scheduling outings for grocery shopping, social outings and exercise are vital aspects of the caregivers' role.

Summary

Management of chronic persistent pain often requires a multidisciplinary approach. Treating the source of the pain condition in addition to all of the physical changes that accompany persistent chronic pain are important. Regular exercise is an essential part of achieving optimal human body function. Non-pharmacological therapies help the patient to start on a journey to improve his/her ability to perform regular exercise, improve posture, and optimize physical function.

References

1. Kisner C, et al. Therapeutic exercise: foundations and techniques. Fa Davis; 2012 Oct8.

2. Méndez-Rebolledo G, et al. Update on the effects of graded motor imagery and mirror therapy on complex regional pain syndrome type 1: A systematic review.J Back Musculoskelet Rehabil.

3. Gattie E, et al. The Effectiveness of Trigger Point Dry Needling for Musculoskeletal Conditions by Physical Therapists: A Systematic Review and Meta-analysis. J Orthop Sports Phys Ther. 2017 Mar;47(3):133-149. doi: 10.2519/jospt.2017.7096. Epub 2017 Feb 3.

4. Patil NJ, et al. A Randomized Trial Comparing Effect of Yoga and Exercises on Quality of Life in among nursing population with Chronic Low Back Pain. Int J Yoga. 2018 Sep-Dec;11(3):208-214.

5. Innes KE, et al. Evid Based Complement Alternat Med. 2018 Aug 30;2018:7683897. Kalauokalani D1, et al. A comparison of physician and nonphysician acupuncture treatment for chronic low back pain. Clin J Pain. 2005 Sep-Oct;21(5):406-11.

6. Wang H, et al. The Most Commonly Treated Acupuncture Indications in the United States: A Cross-Sectional Study. Am J Chin Med. 2018 Oct 9:1-33.

NUTRITION AND PAIN

Introduction

People can have chronic pain for many reasons. It can be muscle pain, nerve pain, joint pain, or other potential types of pain due to cancer, injury or obesity. There are many drugs people use to help treat pain, but often people still do not have adequate control of their pain using these drugs and they may get side effects from the drugs. Since pain can come from many causes and people can respond differently to treatments of pain, using other forms of pain management is often needed. One way to help reduce pain is getting the proper nutrition from your diet. There are also specific nutrients that are believed to help treat pain that will be reviewed in this chapter.

Topic

Pain can be a symptom of many different diseases from cancer to arthritis [1]. The food that you eat can affect how your body feels and can either create or help treat pain. There are some foods that are believed to make pain worse and, some, in turn, that can improve chronic pain control. It is believed that food can cause or make pain worse in many different ways. For example, processed foods have a lot of unhealthy fat, refined sugar, salt, and chemicals, such as pesticides and preservatives. Also, these foods are low in fiber, vitamins, and antioxidants [2]. A diet high in processed foods can make people overweight or obese and can increase inflammation. Obesity is known to increase people's pain [3]. However, food that causes inflammation, or makes inflammation worse, is thought to be the primary reason for causing pain.

Inflammation can be part of many chronic, or long term, pain conditions such as nerve pain [1]. When you get an infection or have an injury, your body tries to help heal itself. It releases substances called "cytokines" from your immune system (the part of your body that reacts to foreign invaders) that start fighting the infection or work to heal the injury [1]. This healing process results in inflammation, which can then cause pain.

Often, once you are healed, the pain and inflammation will go away. Sometimes the inflammation and pain do not go away after your body recovers from the actual injury and this is what commonly causes chronic pain.

Foods that are thought to make inflammation worse are simple carbohydrates, such as white sugar, bread, pastries, processed cereals, white rice or potatoes, fried foods, and red meat [2]. A diet high in any or all these things can worsen inflammation and any pain that is related to the inflammation. This pain can be due to any reason, including nerve pain, joint pain, and fibromyalgia.

Oxidative stress can also result in pain, so use of anti-oxidants, like cherries or olive oil, can improve pain [1]. Use of the Mediterranean diet, which uses the antioxidant rich olive oil as the main source of fat, has been shown to reduce arthritis pain [4].

Just as foods that are highly processed and provide few valuable nutrients, unprocessed, plant- based food can be used as part of the treatment to help treat pain. Some foods that are considered to work against inflammation are green leafy vegetables, avocados, yams, berries, nuts and seeds, lentils and beans, fish (omega-3 oils) and whole grains [2,5].

Food provides both macronutrients and micronutrients. Macro, or large, nutrients are the proteins, carbohydrates and fats in diet. Micro, or small, nutrients are the vitamins, minerals, and antioxidants in food and are found in mostly fresh, unprocessed food.

There are specific diets that are suggested to help with different disease states and pain related to those diseases. The stomach and other parts of the gastrointestinal tract (commonly referred to as gut) are the main areas in the body where substances from the diet get absorbed into the body. If the gut is inflamed, more things can get through, including bacteria and other toxic substances. The immune system lives near the gut and can be triggered to start working if too many bad substances get through the gut wall, creating inflammation [2].

Inflammation of the gut itself can cause pain and gluten free and grain free diets have been tried in irritable bowel syndrome to help reduce pain and inflammation [2]. Gluten is a substance found in breads and pastas. A gluten free diet is necessary for patients who have celiac disease, as they do not have the proper enzymes to break down the grains and become very ill if these are eaten. However, gluten free diets have been used to try and reduce pain associate with migraine and fibromyalgia as well [2]. For the treatment of joint pain and arthritis, a diet that does not contain tomatoes, potatoes, peppers, eggplant and tobacco has been tried.

It is difficult to point out the exact way these diets help with pain control since the studies used to test them are not as strong as studies used to test drugs. This has to do with the fact that changes with diet will take time to show changes in the body and the absorption and use of drugs in the body can be different from person to person [2].

Some of the micronutrients and supplements that are suggested to relieve pain are vitamin D, omega-3 oils, soy, sucrose, vitamin B12, magnesium, and turmeric [1-3,5]. All of these agents are felt to help with nerve pain and/or inflammation.

The body gets vitamin D from the sun. Many people have low vitamin D levels, especially those people who live in areas where sun exposure is limited for a good part of the year, like northern climates. Larger deficiencies in vitamin D have been seen in patients with chronic pain and replacing the vitamin helps to relieve some of the pain. Low vitamin D levels have been associated with inflammation and muscle weakness and can aggravate or cause pain [2,5]. If it is not possible to get enough vitamin D naturally from the sun, a person can take a supplement that is available to buy over the counter.

Omega-3 oils and omega-6 oils are found in diet. A good balance of these is needed for a healthy diet. Often the American diet is too high in omega-6 oils and too low in omega-3 oils. Why is this important to pain? Omega-6 oils can increase inflammation in the body as part of how they work [2]. If we eat too many foods rich in omega-6 oils, we can worsen inflammation and pain. Omega-3 oils work the opposite of omega-6 oils and reduce inflammation and pain [2,5]. Omega-3 oils can be found in flax, fish, free-range eggs, and grass-fed beef [2]. It has been found that omega-3 oils can decrease headache pain and allow patients with rheumatoid arthritis, a specific kind of inflammatory arthritis, to decrease their intake of nonsteroidal ant-inflammatory drugs (NSAIDs), like ibuprofen or naproxen, they were taking and still get pain relief [2,5]. The best source of omega-3 oils are from diet. There are over the counter products that have "fish oils" in them. It is important to read the labels carefully to see what and how much oil is in the capsules. The purest fish oil capsules will have at least half of the listed strength as eicosatetraenoic acid/docosahexaenoic acid (EPA/DHA), which are found in omega-3 acid, with the recommended daily dose being 3000 mg to 4000 mg [2]. There are also prescription products that are omega-3 oils; however, these products are typically used to help lower cholesterol or help prevent heart disease, and none of them are approved for use in the treatment of pain.

Soybeans and soybean oil contain a substance called isoflavones [1]. Isoflavones have several actions on the body, one being anti-inflammatory. Isoflavones can work as estrogens and antioxidants. They can work both centrally in the brain and peripherally, in the nerve endings [1]. When studied in animals, soy helped when given before a painful experience (like surgery) though the pain relief did not last long [1]. There is also proof that soy works in some pain conditions like arthritis and cancer pain, but it can make migraine headaches worse. It also appears that soy is a more effective treatment in men with arthritis than women [3]. It is not currently clear when soy will work in a specific patient with pain.

Sucrose is a sugar and eating this substance has been shown to relieve pain [1]. As an example, when sucrose was given to newborns after they just had a heel stick for a blood draw, crying time was shortened [1]. The way sucrose works is that when you eat it, it changes your body's opioid system and releases substances that are also released when a person is taking opioids, like morphine. By doing this, pain relief is felt. It has also been studied that using sucrose, or another sweet substance, at the same time as morphine, allows morphine to work better. It is not fully understood why this happens and it is unclear if it is due to the sucrose working directly on the morphine to provide more of the drug to the body or if it works on the opioid system in the body in a way that helps morphine work better [1].

A side effect of low B12 levels is chronic pain. It was found that even in pain patients who had normal B12 levels, giving a B12 shot helped improve their pain [2,5].

Magnesium is also an important supplement for the body. It helps with bone formation, and also works on the nerves and helps the muscles relax [2]. By helping these two things, it can help relieve pain from muscle spasms and nerve pain. Fibromyalgia is a type of full body pain with what they call "trigger points" that can be touched to make pain worse. People with fibromyalgia typically have low magnesium levels [6]. Magnesium is also commonly used as a medication to help prevent, when taken every day, or treat, when given once in a while, migraine headaches. When magnesium was used in conjunction with opioids, the effect of the opioids improved, and side effects were reduced [5]. Magnesium is available in oral tablets and solutions. It is often used to treat constipation. Because of this action of the drug, if taking tablets to increase magnesium, it is usually dosed to the point where it can be tolerated without having diarrhea. For the best absorption past the gut, magnesium oxide is often recommended [2]. Magnesium oxide tablets can be purchased over the counter.

Turmeric has more recently become a popular treatment for pain and other ailments. This is a common spice found in the store and is studied for its anti-inflammatory actions. The actual part of turmeric that is felt to relieve pain is curcumin [2,3,5].

Curcumin was found to have the same pain relief as ibuprofen when used for arthritis of your knee [3] and can be used to reduce the need for NSAIDs [5]. It seems that curcumin is best used in the body when cooked or taken with oil and black pepper, making it effective when used in recipes [2]. However, tablets containing curcumin can still be effective and often are much easier to use.

Summary

As many of these small nutrients and vitamins can be purchased over the counter in a pharmacy or nutrition store, it is important to pay attention to the labels on the bottles and make sure they contain the ingredients that you are looking for. Otherwise, getting the proper nutrition from a well-balanced, fresh, non-processed diet, rich in omega-3 oils and nutrients, will likely help treat chronic pain to some degree. The study of nutrition in pain control is limited, but with the move toward a more holistic treatment of pain and reduced use of opioids when able, alternative treatments are needed and can be worth trying.

References

1. Tall JM, et al. Dietary constituents as novel therapies for pain. Clin J Pain. 2004;20(1):19-26.

2. Tick H. Nutrition and pain. Phys Med Rehabil Clin N Am. 2015;26(2):309-320.

3. De Gregori M, et al. Combining pain therapy with lifestyle: the role of personalized nutrition and nutritional supplements according to the SIMPAR Feed Your Destiny approach. J Pain Res. 2016; 9:1179-1189.

4. Veronese N, et al. Adherence to the Mediterranean diet is associated with better quality of life: data from the Osteoarthritis Initiative. Am J Clin Nutr. 2016;104(5):1403-1409.

5. Tick H, et al. Evidence-Based Nonpharmacologic Strategies for Comprehensive Pain Care: The Consortium Pain Task Force White Paper. Explore (NY). 2018;14(3):177-211.

6. Rossi A, et al. Fibromyalgia and nutrition: what news? Clin Exp Rheumatol. 2015;33(1 Suppl 88): S117-125.

MEDICATIONS FOR TREATING CHRONIC PAIN

Introduction

There are many different types of drugs that can be used to treat several different kinds of pain, including nerve pain, muscle pain, joint pain, and cancer pain. They all have different mechanisms of action and often are used together to help control the pain in many ways.

Many of the drugs were originally designed to treat other things like depression and seizures. Some pain disorders, depression and seizures affect the brain and nervous system. Drugs can work for more than one thing just by the way they target different parts of the cells and functions of the body. Having so many kinds of medications to treat pain can be very helpful because chronic pain can be complex and may require several different ways to help relieve the pain and make a person feel more comfortable. Each class of drugs have different side effects that they can cause as well, so having different options can help someone find relief and not have to put up with unnecessary side effects.

The following is a description of several different types of drugs that can help treat pain.

Acetaminophen

Acetaminophen is thought to work on the serotonin receptors to help treat pain. It is also believed it can work on the prostaglandins, similarly to NSAIDs (see below), but does not help inflammation. Serotonin receptors are in the brain and activating these receptors provides both pain relief and improved mood. Acetaminophen is indicated for use to treat fevers and to help relieve minor pains. It is often used as the first medication to treat joint pain, or arthritis. Acetaminophen is well tolerated when taken in correct doses. Patient cannot take over 4 grams of acetaminophen a day on a regular basis as it can build up to toxic levels in the liver and can cause liver failure [1,2].

Nonsteroidal anti-inflammatory agents (NSAIDs)

Nonsteroidal anti-inflammatory agents (NSAIDs) work on cyclooxygenase (COX) receptors and prevent formation of prostaglandins [1,2]. By doing this they exert their pain relief effect by treating inflammation. There are COX1 and COX2 receptors. Depending on how much each one works on each receptor different side effects can occur. All NSAIDs, except celecoxib that is COX2 only, work on both COX1 and COX2 receptors to varying degrees. NSAIDs are routinely used to treat pain associated with inflammation, like joint pain of both osteoarthritis and rheumatoid arthritis. They are also used for acute pain relief for many disorders, including headaches and muscle pain. Examples of NSAIDs include: celecoxib, ibuprofen, naproxen, indomethacin, diclofenac, nabumetone, etodolac, ketorolac, piroxicam, and meloxicam.

Table 1: Adverse events of NSAIDs [2]:

Black box warning*	
Gastrointestinal (GI)	Mild to severe stomach issues.
	Mild: heartburn, pain, diarrhea: happens in up to 40% of people who take NSAIDs.
	Moderate: stomach erosion or ulcers (holes in stomach lining) that are not causing pain/bleeding: happens in up to 30% of people who take NSAIDs.
	Severe: ulcers that are causing pain and/or bleeding: happens
Cardiovascular (Heart Related)	Can cause heart attack, stroke, heart failure, blood clots, and sudden death.
Regular Warnings	
Allergic reactions	Worsening asthma (this is more common with aspirin); rash or itching of the skin, sometimes severe.
Kidney injury	Can cause kidney dysfunction, fluid retention and high blood pressure.

*Black box warning: this is a warning that is issued by the FDA based on available data/information that the drug company must highlight in the drug labeling; it is the highest form of a warning of side effects of a drug.

NSAIDs are very acidic chemicals and can cause stomach ulcers if taken on a regular basis without using a protectant medication, like ranitidine or omeprazole, at the same time. Besides ulcers, NSAIDs have been linked to cardiac risks. As more information becomes available about the side effects, it is not recommended to be on long term NSAIDs unless the benefit they are providing for the pain is more than the risk they are creating by taking them. A list of warnings and possible side effects are listed in the following table.

Some NSAIDs can also be used topically, on the skin, and can be placed at the site of pain [3]. Diclofenac comes in patch and gel forms. Unfortunately, it has not been shown that you can reduce the known side effects from these drugs by using it locally instead of taking it by mouth.

Steroids

Steroid medications can also be used to relieve pain due to inflammation and headaches. They are sometimes used in cancer and radiation related pain. Dexamethasone is preferred for cancer related inflammation pain because you only need to take it once a day [1]. Methylprednisolone is used to treat headaches, but usually only once in a while, not as a daily medication. Because steroids have many side effects, both short term (like stomach upset and irritation, increased appetite, and insomnia) and long term (decrease bone strength, changes in fat placement, weight gain), they are not typically used on a regular basis for pain unless absolutely necessary based on the person's condition.

Antidepressants

Many different antidepressants have been used for treating pain syndromes. The most commonly used antidepressant classes used are tricyclic antidepressants such as amitriptyline and nortriptyline, selective serotonin reuptake inhibitors (SSRIs) such as fluoxetine, and serotonin-norepinephrine reuptake inhibitors (SNRIs) such as duloxetine and venlafaxine. The table below highlights some of the most common antidepressants used for treating pain, some of the uses of these drugs, how they work in the body and side effects that may be experienced [1]. A rare side effect, called serotonin syndrome, can happen when taking too much of any of the listed agents or using them with other drugs that may interact with them. This syndrome can cause agitation, rapid heart rate, incoordination, and nausea/vomiting and can be life threatening [2]. Also, all antidepressants have a black box warning regarding a potential for increase in depression symptoms when people start taking these medications [2].

Table 2: Antidepressants:

Drug	Indications	*Mechanism of action	Common side effect
Tricyclic antidepressants (TCAs)			
Amitriptyline Nortriptyline Imipramine Desipramine	Depression, anxiety, nerve pain, fibromyalgia, sleep and migraine headaches.	Increases action of neurotransmitters (serotonin and norepinephrine) and block sodium channels in the nervous system.	Dry mouth, blurred vision, constipation, low blood pressure and change in heart rhythms.
Selective serotonin reuptake inhibitors (SSRIs)			

Fluoxetine	Depression, binge-eating disorder and fibromyalgia.	Increases serotonin levels.	Nervousness, insomnia, anorexia, nausea and sexual side effects.
Serotonin-norepinephrine reuptake inhibitors (SNRIs)			
Duloxetine Venlafaxine	Depression, nerve pain, fibromyalgia and migraine headaches.	Increases serotonin and norepinephrine.	Low or high blood pressure.

*Mechanism of action: how the drug works in the body; neurotransmitter: a chemical that is released from a nerve fiber and sent to another area (nerve, muscle, etc.).

Anti-seizure medication (anticonvulsants) and sodium-channel blockers

Anti-seizure medications can also be used to help treat nerve pain and headaches. There are different types of anti-seizure medications but the two primary types that help control pain are gamma-aminobutyric acid (GABA) related agents, gabapentin and pregabalin, and sodium channel blockers, carbamazepine, lamotrigine, valproic acid, and topiramate [1,4]. Lidocaine, while not an anti-seizure medication, does block sodium channels and can be used to treat pain [4].

Gabapentin and pregabalin work in a very similar way. Based on their names, you might think they, like the antidepressants listed above, work on GABA receptors. However, they do not. They both resemble GABA in the body, but do not affect the receptors or affect how GABA is treated in the body [1,2]. They actually work on calcium-channels which slows down neurotransmitters and calms nerve pain [1,2]. This same action helps control seizures in people who have a seizure disorder. The main difference between gabapentin and pregabalin is how they are dosed. Gabapentin should be started at a low dose and increased slowly until patient gets the desired effect and limited sided effects [1]. Pregabalin can be started and the dose increased in a quicker time frame as long as the patient can tolerate any side effects they may get [1]. The most common side effects related to both agents are dizziness, drowsiness, fatigue and nausea [2]. The side effects of these drugs tend to go away after a time, so if someone is very tired when first starting the medication, they may need to either reduce the dose and increase more slowly or they need to give their body time to get used to the medication and the side effect may go away.

Other anti-seizure medications work mostly on sodium channels. Extra sodium channels are found in the area when a person have a nerve injury and they also help "excitable" cells to form and create more activity (i.e. pain or seizures) [4]. The most common side effects of these drugs are due to effects on the nervous system, including dizziness and drowsiness. Lamotrigine has caused a severe rash in patients, typically if the dose was started too high or increased too fast. Topiramate also can cause memory or sensory problems in some patients [2].

Lidocaine can be used topically, as a patch or ointment, or it can be used as an infusion. The patches or ointment can be placed on the affected area with pain to help reduce the pain. The patch or ointment can be used alone, but usually they are used along with other medications to help control pain. The patch should be placed on the affected area for 12 hours a day and then removed for 12 hours a day [1,2]. However, it has been found that it is safe to leave the patch on for a full 24 hours if needed. Because lidocaine is also used to put your heart back into a normal rhythm, the doses used to treat pain have been studied in a way to make sure the amount of lidocaine getting into our body does not affect the heart. It was found that up to four patches left on for 12-24 hours a day for 3 full days were safe and well tolerated [1]. Intravenous (in the vein) and subcutaneous (under the skin) lidocaine have also been used to treat pain. This type of therapy requires a person to go into a clinic, infusion center, or hospital to receive therapy. Low-dose intravenous lidocaine infusions given weekly for 4 weeks were found to help decrease nerve pain in some patients [5].

It is important to give the lowest dose possible to try and avoid serious side effects, like irregular heart rhythms. Lidocaine infusions are most commonly used after many other pain treatments have failed or are not working as well as one might want.

Opioids

Opioid medications, or narcotics, are often used in cancer related pain and have been used more frequently in all chronic pain conditions. Opioids work on specific areas in the body called opioid receptors and by attaching to these receptors they affect how you respond to pain and lessen the pain effect [2]. However, opioids can also cause a "high" feeling as they work in the central nervous system, and there is a risk of addiction or dependence on the drugs. Also, the side effects of dizziness, drowsiness, and constipation are all related to the opioids working on the receptors [2]. Constipation occurs because the opioids are also binding to receptors in the gut, which assist in regulating bowel movements. Opioids are available in long-acting products, like oxycodone extended-release (ER), hydrocodone ER, morphine ER, fentanyl patch, and short-acting products, like oxycodone immediate-release (IR), morphine IR, hydrocodone/acetaminophen, and fentanyl lollipops. The two types are often used together to help control pain all day, using the IR tablets as needed to any extra pain you may have. A full review of opioids in the treatment of pain is reviewed in another chapter.

Naltrexone

Naltrexone, at a full dose, actually blocks the opioid receptors [2] and prevents them from working and can make pain worse. Interestingly, at low doses, naltrexone works differently and is thought to attach to other receptors in the nervous system and reduce inflammation [6,7]. Current literature discussed the use of low dose naltrexone for patients with pain due to multiple sclerosis, fibromyalgia, and Crohn's disease [6,7]. However, there is information suggesting it works in many other kinds of nerve pain as well. There are no noted side effects from therapy outside of opioid withdrawal, which occurs with regular strength doses [6,7]. Naltrexone for opioid dependence is dosed starting at 50 mg, whereas low-dose naltrexone typically ranges from 1 mg to 5 mg [6,7]. All low dose naltrexone preparations need to be compounded by a pharmacist because it is not commercially available in the small doses.

Benzodiazepines

Benzodiazepine drugs include lorazepam, alprazolam, temazepam, diazepam and clonazepam, among others. Use of these drugs is typically for treatment of anxiety and muscle spasm. They can also be used for sleep and seizures. Benzodiazepines work on the GABA receptors and enhance GABA activity and slow down neurotransmitters. The time it takes different benzodiazepines to work in your system and how fast the effect goes away varies for each agent. That is why they are used for different reasons in clinical practice. Lorazepam and diazepam are used in fast seizure control and clonazepam, because it can be taken once a day and work all day, may be used to help control seizures from starting. Temazepam is used for sleep; other agents are not recommended as sleeping agents. Clonazepam is also used for anxiety, as are lorazepam and alprazolam; however, lorazepam and alprazolam work quickly and stop working earlier, and are not used on a regular basis to treat anxiety. Lorazepam and diazepam are sometimes used to help prevent muscle spasms. Prevention of muscle spasms can help relieve pain. Because of how it works, clonazepam has been looked at for pain control and may be effective in some cases. Benzodiazepines can cause drowsiness, dizziness, and slow your breathing. When used with opioids, these effects can be worse as they have an additive effect. It is not recommended to take benzodiazepines with opioids, but if needed, then doctor will help find the right doses and closely monitor the patient [2].

Muscle Relaxants

There are drugs that decrease muscle spasms due to painful conditions and some that reduce spasms due to diseases that cause increase in muscle tone (spasticity), such as cerebral palsy [1]. Most muscle relaxants are used for short term pain relief; however, others may be used longer, especially when treating chronic spasticity. Drugs that are considered muscle relaxants and are not benzodiazepines are cyclobenzaprine, orphenadrine, metaxalone, carisoprodol, tizanidine and baclofen. All muscle relaxants show their effects in the brain and central nervous system and reduce activity to help slow down firing to the muscles and reduce spasms [1,2]. The drugs have been shown to work in relieving spasms and pain associated with the spasms, however, they have significant side effects, particularly severe drowsiness, that can limit their use [1,2]. Some of them, like cyclobenzaprine and orphenadrine cause dry mouth and constipation. The following table lists some muscle relaxants and their common side effects.

Table 3: Muscle relaxants [1,2]:

Drug	Common Side Effect
Cyclobenzaprine	Drowsiness, dizziness, and dry mouth.
Orphenadrine	Drowsiness, dizziness, dry mouth, and increased heart rate.
Metaxalone	Drowsiness, dizziness, and nausea.
Carisoprodol	Drowsiness, and dizziness.
Tizanidine	Drowsiness, dizziness, dry mouth, and low blood pressure.
Baclofen	Drowsiness, confusion, decrease muscle tone, headache, nausea, and vomiting.

All the medications can be given by mouth, but baclofen is also available to be used in a spinal pump for patients with severe spasticity.

Summary

There are many different options to treat pain. Treatment of the individual patient will depend on where their pain is coming from, how long they have had the pain, what has already been used to treat the pain, and how well they tolerate the side effects of the different medications. Because the body and nervous system are complex, the actions of some drugs used to treat other disorders, like depression and seizures, are commonly used and have shown benefit in the treatment of pain disorders. By having all the available options, hopefully a person's specific pain can be targeted with the most appropriate therapies.

There is always ongoing work to look at new treatments or new ways to use treatments we currently have to help better treat chronic pain.

References

1. Wickham RJ. Cancer Pain Management: Comprehensive Assessment and Nonopioid Analgesics, Part 1. J Adv Pract Oncol. 2017;8(5):475-490.

2. Lexicomp Online, Lexi-Drugs: Wolters Kluwer Clinical Drug Information, Inc.; 2018; October 25, 2018.

3. Derry S et al. Topical NSAIDs for chronic musculoskeletal pain in adults. Cochrane Database Syst Rev. 2016;4:CD007400.

4. Kalso E. Sodium channel blockers in neuropathic pain. Curr Pharm Des.2005;11(23):3005-3011.

5. Kim YC, et al. Efficacy and Safety of Lidocaine Infusion Treatment for Neuropathic Pain: A Randomized, Double-Blind, and Placebo-Controlled Study. Reg Anesth Pain Med. 2018;43(4):415-424.

6. Patten DK, et al. The Safety and Efficacy of Low-Dose Naltrexone in the Management of Chronic Pain and Inflammation in Multiple Sclerosis, Fibromyalgia, Crohn's Disease, and Other Chronic Pain Disorders. Pharmacotherapy. 2018;38(3):382- 389.

7. Toljan K, et al. Low-Dose Naltrexone (LDN)-Review of Therapeutic Utilization. Med Sci (Basel). 2018;6(4).

PROCEDURES FOR TREATING CHRONIC PAIN

Introduction

To say chronic pain is a challenge is a major understatement! It can be a constant hardship for those who face it personally, the friends and family who support them through it, and the practitioners who manage it. During certain instances in the management of chronic pain, medications, physical therapy, and behavioral therapy may fail to provide substantial pain relief or adequate improvement in functionality. In these instances, more invasive procedures (invasive meaning the introduction of instruments into the body) may be of benefit.

There is a large list of procedures that can be used to treat many different causes of pain in various areas of the body. Different techniques utilize distinct devices and medications. Each procedure is specifically suited to decrease discomfort and improve functionality in the area in which the person experiences pain. Commonly, such as for those individuals with chronic back pain, a clear source of pain may not be present or multiple sources may exist. In those circumstances, physicians attempt to identify the highest probable source or the most painful area to target first. Sometimes multiple interventions or different types of interventions may need to be performed for the patient to see a benefit.

Regardless of the specific technique, each procedure is only one part of a multimodal (multiple methods) treatment regimen for the management of pain. As stated before, the goal of any chronic pain procedure is to decrease pain and improve functionality; an individual procedure may not eliminate all pain. When these techniques are successful, it is still extremely important for individuals to continue to focus on other parts of the treatment plan such as proper diet, exercise, physical therapy, behavior modification, and medication management to increase the duration and effectiveness of the chronic pain procedure.

It can be extremely stressful when conservative therapies for chronic pain have not provided significant relief. Physicians realize that needing to consider an invasive procedure for the next step in pain management can be troubling to those suffering from chronic pain.

Furthermore, numerous questions and concerns may arise from patients and their families alike. It is one of the most important jobs of a physician to explain, teach, and to make sure the patient is informed since everyone learns at their own pace.

This chapter will thoroughly discuss chronic pain procedures. We will explain the reasons why physicians use certain chronic pain procedures, how the procedures are performed, and the risks associated with each procedure. We will begin by defining the medications used in each procedure and their purpose. Next, specific procedures will be outlined including intraarticular and periarticular joint injections, epidural steroid injections, and medial branch blocks. We will describe the risks, benefits, and expectations of each procedure. We will also discuss important safety precautions such as what to do when patients are on anticoagulation or antibiotics. The goal of this chapter is to answer common questions to eliminate fear revolving around chronic pain procedures and to provide patients and those who support patients an increased understanding as to what occurs the day of the procedure.

Medications

The two types of medications which comprise the cornerstone of most chronic pain procedures are local anesthetics and corticosteroids. During the majority of chronic pain procedures local anesthetics are used to numb the area of the body into which the corticosteroids will be deposited. The goal is to place the power of anti-inflammatory steroids at the primary site of inflammation thus decreasing pain and improving a patient's experience. In addition, local anesthetics can be used to block a nerve. There are other drugs which can be used during these procedures such is antibacterial cleansers, contrast dye and pain/sedation medications that can improve patient comfort during the chronic pain procedure itself. Each will be discussed in detail in the following section.

Corticosteroids

Corticosteroids may be the single most important medications in chronic pain procedures. This type of medication has been in existence since the 1940s and simulates cortisone-like hormones that your body naturally produces to maintain your health. These are powerful drugs that decrease inflammation by multiple mechanisms such as preventing the release of inflammatory substances by white blood cells, decreasing blood vessel permeability to eliminate swelling, and acting as an anti-histamine. Less inflammation means less neuronal irritation (irritation of the nerves) which is commonly transmitted to the brain as pain signals.

There are a variety of steroid medications currently on the market. Each medication has its own unique features, potency, and side effects which will be considered by a physician before use. It is estimated that the steroid injection takes approximately 2-3 days to begin working and up to 2-3 weeks for the patient to see the full benefit. The duration of the effect is unique to each patient based on the cause of pain, the amount of inflammation, and the response of the patient to the drug. That is why in many procedures, providers will add a local anesthetic to steroids. Local anesthetics will have a fast onset but a short duration of action. The goal is to have pain relief by the local anesthetics until the effect of steroids kicks in.

While steroids are naturally produced in the body and are usually well-tolerated, they do pose some potential side effects, most of which occur with long-term administration. The most common side effect of localized steroid injections is swelling in the feet or hands due to increased fluid retention. Though uncommon, steroids can cause an exacerbation of congestive heart failure in individuals with cardiac disease [1]. Also, increased blood sugar can be provoked especially in those individuals with diabetes. Other side effects such as increased blood pressure, nervousness, headache, and allergic reactions are very rare. Commonly, physicians limit the number of steroid injections you can receive to no more than once every 6 weeks and no more than 4 injections per year, though this may vary. If you have diabetes, heart disease or kidney disease, or issues with steroids in the past, it is important to discuss this with your pain management team.

Local Anesthetics

The first local anesthetic was created over 100 years ago and has been a significant tool in the treatment of pain. The word anesthesia means loss of sensation, thus individuals who are injected with these medications report a sense of numbness in the area of the injection. Local anesthetics work by preventing the ability of a nerve to transmit pain signals on its surface. The most commonly utilized local anesthetic during chronic pain procedures is lidocaine, but other longer-lasting medications such as ropivacaine and bupivacaine can also be used during certain procedures.

Local anesthetics can be injected for two purposes. The first and most common purpose is to provide a painless area to perform the procedure. This is done by injecting the skin and underlying tissue with the medication immediately before the procedure. The injection of the local anesthetic itself may present with a burning sensation, commonly described as a "bee sting". This sensation usually lasts for less than 10 seconds and is then replaced by numbness. The second purpose of local anesthetics in chronic pain procedures is to identify and diagnose the source(s) of pain. Local anesthetics can also be injected in a hypothesized source of pain such as a joint or tissue. If the pain improves, a physician can assume this is the source of pain and according provide a more precise diagnosis. This can lead to more target pain interventions in the future which will be discussed in later chapters.

Local anesthetics are some of the most widely utilized medications and have very limited side effects. Concern with local anesthetics is primarily related to the amount of drug injected and whether patients have allergies to these medications. The dose of local anesthetics used in chronic pain procedures is far less than any toxic level. For individuals who have had reactions to local anesthetics in the past, it is vital that you discuss this with your physicians as there are different classes of local anesthetics which can be avoided or substituted.

Skin Cleanser

Some may not think of skin cleanser or soap as a type of medication, but it is included here briefly to be sure individuals reading this chapter know everything that they will experience during a chronic pain procedure. The two main types of skin cleansers are iodine and chlorohexidine in alcohol. In recent years, chlorohexidine has been employed more frequently due to its enhanced bacterial killing abilities [2]. In terms of deciding which cleanser to use, be sure to inform your physician if you have any history of allergic reactions, as this the greatest factor in choosing a specific cleanser.

Radiographic Contrast

Another substance that may be employed if your injection is being guided by fluoroscopy (x-ray) is a contrast agent. Contrast is used in certain injections to determine whether the needle is in the correct position. Essentially, contrast media is injected via a syringe and a picture is taken under fluoroscopy. Contrast flows in a different fashion depending on the specific tissue area or if it is accidently placed into a blood vessel; it allows another way for the physician completing the pain procedure to ensure he/she is placing the medication in the right place. There are multiple types of contrast, but all are iodine-based. They have minimal side effects, but if the patient has had a prior reaction to iodine, including an allergic reaction or anaphylaxis, they should inform their physician as it may be best to avoid contrast all together.

Opioids and Sedatives

Typically, injection of a local anesthetic during chronic pain procedures causes minimal discomfort. In individuals who struggle with severe pain or have anxiety during the procedure, small doses of short-acting opioids and/or benzodiazepines (such as fentanyl and midazolam) may be given. These medications require the placement of an intravenous catheter (IV) for administration. If given, the patient is closely monitored for side effects such as respiratory depression and hypotension. Providers have different preference when it comes to the administration of those medications during a procedure. Further discussion of these medication is beyond the scope of this chapter.

Chronic Pain Procedures

In our exploration of the chronic pain procedures it is important to first understand what types of injections exist and why they are performed. There are many complicated words surrounding chronic pain procedures such as periarticular, interarticular, cervical, and medial branch. These terms can seem like a foreign language and have no relative meaning to those individuals who are not trained in medicine or pain management. Thus, as we explore each type of injection, it will be important to define some basic terms in order have a foundation on which to build our understanding of chronic pain procedures. After which we will discuss the procedure itself and the benefits/risks.

Joint Injections

Structure of a Joint and Terminology

To begin, let's review general terms surrounding joint injections. A joint is a portion of the body where two or more bones come together. Joints allow for movement and are commonly supported by ligaments which are short bands of strong and flexible connective tissue that connect the bones together. A common example would be the anterior cruciate ligament, more commonly referred to as the "ACL" which prevents excessive movement of the bones at your knee. Ligaments act like a hinge allowing the bones to pivot next to one another. Tendons, on the other hand, are the connective tissue that attaches muscles to bones. Like ligaments, they are strong, but they provide a different function. They act as attachments between muscle and bones and thus provide movement; they are essentially the pulleys of the body, pulling bones along as the muscles contract. A common tendon is the Achilles tendon which connects the muscles of your calf to the base of your foot. This allows individuals to stand on their tiptoes. If the tendon ruptures a person will have decrease ability to move their foot at the ankle, support weight on their ankle, and point their toes at the floor.

The last two portions of joints that are usually discussed are the joint capsule and bursa. The capsule is essentially the cushion or "shock absorber" in the joint. It is composed of strong cartilage on the outside and thick synovial fluid on the inside. The synovial fluid acts like a lubricant and cushions the joint from the repetitive force it endures throughout our life as we move. Bursas, the final part of the joint, act like padding to cushion the muscles and prevent them from becoming worn down. For example, if you were to lift a heavy object into a high floor of a building using a rope, you would not want to pull the rope along a brick windowsill. As you lifted the object, the brick would wear at the rope and cause it to snap. If you think of the rope as a muscle and the brick as a bone, the same would happen in the human body. The bursa of the joint essentially acts like a pulley so that the two surfaces slide past each other, allowing the muscle to slide easily past the bone.

As you may now realize, a joint is a complex structure. It has multiple components, all of which can become damaged resulting in chronic pain. A detailed physical exam and imaging are sometimes needed to diagnose the cause of chronic pain. Once the diagnosis is made different types of joint injections exist to target the different problem areas. When a practitioner places a needle into the interior of the joint (known as the joint capsule), it is commonly referred to as an intraarticular joint injection. When medication is injected near the joint (such as into a bursa or near inflamed ligaments/tendons), it is known as a periarticular injection [3]. The goal in both types of injections is to identify the source of pain and to decrease inflammation. This will likely translate into decreased pain and improved functionality.

Stepwise Description of Joint Injections

Joint injections can be performed under direct visualization, ultrasound-guidance, or fluoroscopy (x-ray). Certain joints are readily assessible via assessment of the relevant anatomy. This is sometimes referred to as a "blind approach" since no imaging is necessary to identify the structure(s). Regardless of the approach, similar steps are used for the procedure. The patient is brought into the procedure room and the joint being injected is marked. A time- out is performed which identifies the patient, the injection site, the patient's allergies, and all other relevant information needed to perform the injection. Next, the area around the joint is prepped with cleaning solution under sterile conditions. This step is extremely important as it helps to decrease risk of infection.

Following proper cleaning and set-up, the joint being injected is assessed by the practitioner by palpation (feeling over the joint to identify the structures) or by using imaging such as ultrasound or x-ray. It may take a few moments for palpation or for multiple images to identify the ideal injection site. Following proper identification, a small amount of local anesthetic, usually lidocaine, is injected into the skin and underlying tissue to provide a numb or painless section. As stated before, local anesthetics are very good for decreasing sharp, stabbing-type pain, however, the patient may still feel pressure during the joint injection. If the individual feels any sharpness during the injection, additional local anesthetic can be injected to provide further pain relief.

Following the creation of a numb or pain-free area, a second (slightly larger) needle is advanced through the prior anesthetized area. The needle is advanced to the planned injection area either within the joint itself (intraarticular) or near the joint (periarticular). Upon reaching the desired area, the physician uses a syringe to confirm the correct location. Sometimes this is also confirmed by x-ray. Once the correct location is identified, the medication is injected. This commonly is a combination of a steroid with or without additional local anesthetic. Once the medication is completely injected the needle is removed, a quick assessment for bleeding at the site is performed, and a bandage is placed over the entry point.

Risk involved with joint injections

The risks involved with joint injections are usually very minimal. Any time anyone breaks the skins protective barrier there is a small chance of infection or bleeding. As previously discussed, sterilizing soap is applied at an attempt to kill all harmful bacteria. The doctor doing the injection also uses knowledge of anatomy and/or imaging to avoid all major blood vessels.

Though rare, with prolonged use of steroids, some patients have thinning of skin/bones near the injection. One of the most common experiences reported by individuals receiving injections is a short period of worsening pain or swelling following the procedure. This experience usually lasts less than 1-2 days and it is extremely important that you inform your physician if you have any adverse reaction following the injection.

Epidural Steroid Injections

Structure of the Epidural Space and Terminology

As we transition to our next injection type, epidural steroid injection, we should again review a few general terms. The epidural space is the area directly behind the spinal cord as it runs through the bony structures that makes up your spine. The two areas are separated by the dural sac which keeps the spinal cord and its protective cerebral spinous fluid on one side and the fatty cushion known as the epidural space on the other. The epidural space is a target for chronic pain injections as it can be safely accessed, allows for medication placement, and follows tissue planes that allow medication to reach inflamed nerve roots above, below, and lateral to the injection site.

There are specific terms which are used to discuss the source of a patient's pain. In general, the term cervical refers to a person's neck. Thoracic describes the mid-back where the vertebrae (back bones) attach to an individual's ribs. Lumbar stands for the low back, and caudal refers to where the epidural space is accessed through the bones that make up the middle of your pelvis. Each area can be targeted specifically based on the source of a person's pain. In addition, you may hear the terms interlaminar or transforaminal when discussing epidural injections. These refer to different access point for epidural injections depending on the area of pain, the source of pain, and the amount of space available within the epidural space itself. Interlaminar describes access to the epidural space in the middle line between the bones, whereas transforaminal describes entering the epidural space on the side of the bone where the nerves leaving the spine exit. The site of the epidural is chosen uniquely by each physician based on a patient's symptoms and pathology to provide the best pain relief for that patient.

Stepwise Description of Epidural Injections

For chronic pain, a patient's epidural injections are commonly performed under fluoroscopy (x-ray). This allows the physician to have an improved assessment of the relevant structures. Regardless of the area or type of epidural injection (interlaminar versus transforaminal) the steps of the procedure are similar. Just as with joint injections, the patient is first brought into a procedure room. The area over the injection site is marked and a time-out is performed which identifies the patient, allergies, and all other relevant information needed to perform the injection. Lastly, the area of skin over the epidural space is prepped with cleaning solution under sterile conditions.

Following proper cleaning and set up, images are taken to determine the proper entrance site for the injection. A local anesthetic is injected into the skin to provide a numb or painless section to perform the procedure. Again, local anesthetics are very good at decreasing sharp, stabbing-type pain, but the patient may still feel pressure during the injection. Using imaging, the epidural needle is advanced carefully to the planned injection site and confirmed to be in proper position using multiple techniques. Before any injection, the physician uses a contrast dye to make sure that the needle is not inside a blood vessel and has not traveled too far forward into the cerebrospinous fluid. Once the epidural needle is confirmed to be in the desired area, a steroid with or without local anesthetic is injected. Once the medication is completely injected, the needle is removed, a quick assessment for bleeding at the site is performed, and a bandage is placed over the entry site.

Risk involved with joint injections

The risks of epidural steroid injections are minimal. Due to the puncture of skin, there is again a small chance of infection and bleeding. This risk is decreased with proper pre-operative cleaning techniques. The physician performing the procedure uses the smallest needle(s) possible and/or imaging techniques to avoid damage to surrounding blood vessels. The risk of serious injection or bleeding is less than 0.1% but may require more advanced care due to proximity to the spinal cord [5,6]. Epidural injections have unique risks. Even though these risks are rare, they come with great concern if complications occur. If the dural sac is punctured during the procedure, the cerebrospinal fluid will leak and a post-dural puncture headache may occur. This type of headache is usually worse upon standing due to changes in pressure in the cerebrospinal fluid. Generally, this headache improves within a few days, but sometimes an additional procedure (called a blood patch) may be necessary to decrease headache severity.

Lastly, while cases of nerve injury are exceeding rare, damage may occur during the procedure or from infection or bleeding.

The patient may report a short period of worsening pain and/or swelling following the procedure. This usually lasts less than 1-2 days and is due to placing the medication in an already inflamed area. As always, it is extremely important that you inform your physician if you have any adverse reaction following the injection, especially if you have changes in strength or bowel/bladder function.

Medial Branch Nerve Blocks

Structure of the Epidural Space and Terminology

In describing medial branch nerve blocks (MBB) it is important to define what the medial branch nerve is and what it provides sensation to. The medial branch nerve innervates the facet joint (also sometimes known as zygapophyseal or apophyseal joints). The facet joints are a pair of small joints in the posterior spine that allow the two vertebrae (the bones of the spine) to connect and move in relation to each other. These joints allow us to rotate, flex, and extend our spines safely to prevent too much or too little motion. Over time these joints can become inflamed and worn which translates into pain in our neck or back that does not radiate into our extremities. The medial branch nerve is the nerve that transmits these pain signals. The facet joint is innervated by two different medial branch nerve branches, one from the level of the joint and one from the level above the joint. Thus, multiple sites are injected to block multiple nerves that are likely transmitting the pain signals. By blocking the nerves, physicians can accomplish two goals: 1. verify that this is the source of patient's pain and 2. provide temporary pain relief. Medial branch blocks are used as diagnostic predictors of the efficacy of radiofrequency lesioning (damaging of the nerve) which can provide prolonged back relief. This will be discussed in detail in another chapter.

Stepwise Description of Medial Branch Block

As with epidural steroid injections, MBBs are performed under fluoroscopy (x-ray). This allows the physician an improved assessment of relevant structures. These blocks can be performed on either side of the spine and throughout its entire length. The patient will be brought to a procedure room and the area over the injection site will be marked. A time out is performed which identifies the patient, allergies, and all other relevant information needed to perform the injection. Lastly, the area of skin over the epidural space is prepped with cleaning solution under sterile conditions.

Following proper cleaning and set up, images are taken to determine the proper entrance site for injections. Local anesthetic is injected into the skin to provide a numb or painless section to perform the injection. Compared to the prior discussed injections, multiple areas of skin will need to be anesthetized to provide full coverage for the different sites of the medial branches. Using imaging, the spinal needle is advanced carefully to the planned injection site and confirmed to be in the proper position using multiple technique including taking images at different angles. Once the needle is confirmed to be in the desired area, additional local anesthetic is injected to directly numb the nerve. Once the medication is completely injected, the needle is quickly removed. This process will be completed at each site/level to block the medial branches innervating a specific facet joint(s).

Risks involved with joint injections

Complications from medial branch blocks are exceedingly rare and include infection, bleeding, and nerve injury. Physicians undergo the same steps previously described with epidural injections to attempt to prevent these complications. Unlike previous injections, patient usually report timely relief of their pain if the injection provide benefit. The relief of the pain is usually temporary, lasting the duration of the local anesthetic injected. If the patient receives relief with the injection, then the blocks may be repeated to confirm the benefit, and radiofrequency nerve ablation may follow to provide long-lasting relief.

Anticoagulation/Antibiotics

It is extremely important for individuals who have bleeding disorders or who are using anticoagulation medications (blood thinners) to inform their physician. Commonly used blood thinning medication includes aspirin, Coumadin (warfarin), Plavix (clopidogrel), heparin, or Non-Steroidal Anti-inflammatory Drugs (NSAIDS) (such as ibuprofen or naproxen). In addition, anyone using herbal supplements should tell their doctor as these may have blood-thinning properties [8]. These medications may increase your risk of bleeding and bleeding related side effects. Many of the anticoagulation medications will need to be stopped prior to the procedure to decrease these risks. A conversation between the provider prescribing the blood thinning medication, the pain physician, and the patient will help determine the risks and benefits specific to the patient. In addition, a decision will need to be made as to the duration of time prior to the procedure in which the medication should be stopped and then restarted.

A question commonly asked by the patient undergoing chronic pain procedure is whether they need antibiotics to prevent infection before/after the procedure. To date, there is no research demonstrating routine use of antibiotic for pain procedures [7]. In patients who are at increased risk of infection such as those that are immunocompromised, this discussion will be individual-specific. It is extremely important for those who have had fevers, antibiotic treatment, illnesses, or hospitalization within the last four weeks to discuss this with the physician performing the procedure. It is crucial that the patient be healthy on the day of the procedure.

General Facts

To judge the effectiveness of the chronic pain procedures, the patient should be experiencing their pain symptoms on the day of the procedure. This allows the patient and the physician the ability to determine the benefit of the intervention. The patient should keep a written log of his/her pain scores and activity following the procedure. At some institutions, these logs are completed for a minimum of two weeks. The log becomes a valuable resource for comparison of how the procedure affected the patient's life in terms of pain and functionality and can provide crucial information regarding the benefit of repeat injections in the future.

Other procedures

There are many other procedures performed for chronic pain, we discussed in this chapter the most common ones. Other procedures such as abdominal wall injections, nerve blocks for pain in the head, extremities and pelvis and sympathetic nerve blocks for certain pain conditions, follow the same concepts as described in this chapter.

Summary

It can be stressful when conservative therapies for chronic pain have not provided significant pain relief. A variety of procedures exist to treat pain in various areas of the body. Each is suited to decrease discomfort and improve functionality in the area in which the person experiences pain. Through a complete history, physical exam, and imaging modalities, a pain management physician can specifically tailor chronic pain procedural plan to diagnosis and treat a patient's pain. This chapter aimed to describe common chronic pain procedures and the medications involved to increase patient knowledge and alleviate concerns.

Reference

1. Buenaventura, R., et al. Systematic review of therapeutic lumbar transforaminal epidural steroid injections. Pain Physician 12.1 (2009): 233-251.

2. Darouiche, R., et al. Chlorhexidine–alcohol versus povidone–iodine for surgical-site antisepsis." New England Journal of Medicine 362.1 (2010): 18-26.

3. Peterson C, Hodler, J. Adverse events from diagnostic and therapeutic joint injections: a literature review. Skeletal radiology 40.1 (2011): 5-12.

4. Renfrew, Donald L., et al. Correct placement of epidural steroid injections: fluoroscopic guidance and contrast administration. American Journal of Neuroradiology 12.5 (1991): 1003-1007.

5. Kindler, C., et al. Epidural abscess complicating epidural anesthesia and analgesia: an analysis of the literature. Acta anaesthesiologica scandinavica 42.6 (1998): 614-620.

6. Wulf, H. Epidural anesthesia and spinal hematoma. Canadian Journal of Anesthesia. (1996)4.

7. Epstein NE. The risks of epidural and transforaminal steroid injections in the Spine: Commentary and a comprehensive review of the literature. Surgical neurology international. 2013;43.12 (1996): 1260-1271.

8. Ernst E. Harmless herbs? A review of the recent literature. American Journal of Medicine. 1998; 104:170.

ADVANCED PROCEDURES FOR TREATING CHRONIC PAIN

Introduction

Advanced pain procedures are often necessary for patients to help alleviate their pain and return to a reasonable level of function when conservative measures and basic procedures have failed These procedures can reduce pain and allow patients to return to their day to day activities. Undergoing an invasive procedure can be daunting to patients and their families.

Often times the fear lies in the unfamiliarity of the pre-operative, post-operative, and follow-up instructions as well as the possible adverse events associated with each procedure. The purpose of this chapter is to educate patients regarding the different advanced pain procedures commonly performed by physicians and their indications.

Advanced pain procedures are typically image-guided, either via ultrasound or fluoroscopy, to help with real-time needle localization. Use of an ultrasound poses no radiation risk to the patient, as it uses sound waves at frequencies higher than the upper limit of human hearing to create black and white images [1]. On the other hand, fluoroscopy also known as a portable x-ray, uses radiation transmission to create images. Thus, standard radiation safety and precautions are required. The actual radiation dose differs for each type of procedure and the obstacles that may arise during the procedure. To minimize the radiation risk, physicians traditionally perform the intervention using the lowest acceptable exposure for the shortest time necessary. A typical procedure with no complications exposes the patient to less radiation than a chest x-ray [1]. Pregnant women should notify the physicians immediately as fluoroscopy and medications used during those procedures may have harmful effects on the fetus.

Radiofrequency Ablation

A common type of advanced procedure performed by pain physicians is radiofrequency ablation (RFA). This procedure utilizes a probe inserted inside of large bore needle to send an electric current to heat up the nearby nerve to decrease transmission of pain. RFA is indicated for pain associated with arthritis (neck, back, shoulder, hip, knee), and different nerve conditions all over the body. Usually, patients can expect anywhere from 6-12 months of relief and sometimes more. RFA is a relatively safe procedure with very few complications. Some complications that can occur are bleeding, infection, nerve damage, superficial skin burn and nerve regeneration [1].

Cryoablation

An advanced pain procedure very similar to RFA is cryoablation. Instead of heating the nerve to decrease pain signals, cryoablation freezes the nerve using nitrous oxide gas to decrease pain signals. Cryoablation is indicated for post-thoracotomy pain, lumbar facet syndrome, trigeminal neuralgia, post-herpetic neuralgia, atypical facial pain, Morton's Neuroma, perianal pain, rectal pain, pregnancy-related and post-partum pain, post inguinal herniorrhaphy pain, and various neuralgias and nerve conditions [1]. Complications associated with this procedure can range from neuroma formation, nerve regeneration, neuropathic pain, and local tissue injury with numbness in the involved nerve territory [1]. Some research has reported depigmentation and hair loss at site of lesioning, but this is extremely uncommon.

Preoperative and Postoperative instructions for RFA and Cryoablation

Preoperatively, 6 days prior to the procedure patients should stop aspirin and 5-7 days prior for clopidogrel. For 1 day prior, patients should not take any Ibuprofen or diclofenac and 4 days prior for naproxen (NSAIDs). Anticoagulants such as rivaroxaban and apixaban should be stopped 3 days prior to the procedure. Enoxaparin should be stopped 12 hours prior to the procedure. Patients on warfarin should discuss the risk and benefits with the prescribing physician and the potential need for bridging therapy as it needs to be stopped 5 days with INR<1.2 on the day of the procedure. Patients may resume their scheduled medications 24 hours after the procedure, except warfarin which may be resumed as early as 6 hours postoperatively but ideally the following day (please discuss this with the prescribing physician) and clopidogrel can be resumed in 12 hours. Enoxaparin can be resumed 12-24 hours after the procedure (please confirm with prescribing physician) [2].

Anticoagulation guidelines can change from year to year, so it is imperative for patients to inform their physician about the type of anticoagulant they are prescribed and the reason for its use prior to scheduling and undergoing the procedure. Occasionally, stopping an anticoagulant is not safe and, in that case, physicians may use a bridging protocol where short acting agent is used and can be stopped shortly before procedure and then started shortly after procedure. Afterwards, patients will be bridged to their original anticoagulation medication.

Sometimes even bridging may not be recommended, which can lead to the necessary delay of the procedure until the condition is stabilized. Failure to follow these directions or notifying your physician of medications can lead to cancellation of procedure, increased risk for bleeding, stroke or pulmonary embolism.

If sedation is being used for the procedure, the patient is instructed to refrain from eating or drinking for a set period of time prior to its start. Typically, this is 8 hours for a meal and 2 hours for clear liquids. It is important to discuss these guidelines with your physician as the time depends nature of the drink and meal. For example, a patient may be able to drink water for up to 2 hours before the procedure. Failure to follow these instructions can lead to significant gastrointestinal symptoms such as nausea and vomiting which could potentially be aspirated into the lungs, leading to infection or serious respiratory complications. Post-operatively, patients can expect mild bleeding and bruising in the area, in addition to discomfort and swelling at the site. Ice can be used in cycles of 20 minutes on and 20 minutes off for control of swelling and discomfort for the first 24 hours [3]. Afterwards, patients are recommended to use heat, if better tolerated. Once the local anesthetic has worn off, it is expected for the pain to worsen. Thus, acetaminophen may be used for pain control. Patients may take their pain medications as ordered by their physicians if available. It should be expected that it can often take anywhere from 1-4 weeks for full pain relief [3]. There may be mild weakness postoperatively and thus activity limitation should be followed for the first 2-3 days after the procedure. It is recommended for patients to avoid baths or soaking of the sites for few days [3], but patients can resume showering in 24- 48 hours. Follow-up is at discretion of the physician, but normally patients can follow up once their pain returns to pre-procedure levels or sooner if any complications arise.

Spinal Cord Stimulators

Spinal cord stimulator (SCS) trials and implants are performed at a well-equipped clinic, ambulatory surgery center or an operating room of a hospital due to its advanced nature.

Patients will need to undergo thorough pain and mental health evaluation to qualify for a SCS trial. Additionally, permanent SCS implants require a successful 5-7-day trial with a temporary implant. Before the procedure, patients are commonly prescribed prophylactic antibiotics for infection prevention. The procedure involves a small incision at the midline back to help the physician thread the two stimulator leads into the posterior epidural space of the thoracic or cervical spinal column. Once in the correct position, the patient will be awakened to confirm coverage over area of pain. If the patient successfully passed the trial, a permanent implant is placed with a few minor changes including an additional incision for a battery implantation. SCS initially requires close monitoring with the physician and device representative for troubleshooting and programming. SCS is often indicated for patients with failed back surgery syndrome, chronic radicular pain, neuropathic pain, complex regional pain syndrome, peripheral ischemia, or angina [4].

Complications associated with SCS range from minor problems such as lack of pain coverage or headaches to more severe (very rare) complications such as paralysis, nerve injury, and death [4]. More common complications were found to be lead migration or breakage and infection. A deeper infection can lead to an abscess formation which can lead to paralysis and death if not identified quickly. Serious complications are less likely to occur, but the most reported complication is lead migration which can be addressed by reprogramming the device or performing another minor procedure to place the leads back in their intended location.

Intrathecal Pumps

Implanted drug delivery systems for chronic pain have been around since the 1800s. The goal of implanted drug delivery systems such as intrathecal (IT) pump implants is to achieve superior or similar pain relief as oral medications but without the side effects. Only certain medications such as morphine, baclofen, and ziconotide are approved by the FDA for use in implanted drug delivery systems. Some other medications such as fentanyl and hydromorphone are used off label with good efficacy. It is important for physicians to discuss different options with patients. There are stringent selection criteria determined by the physician that must be met in order to proceed with IT therapy. Like SCS, this procedure is commonly performed in a more monitored setting such as ambulatory surgery center or operating room of a hospital. The IT pump trial is performed either by placing a catheter infusing the drug for 1-2 days which usually requires hospital admission or as a single injection and discharging patient home. In both approaches, patient will report their pain scores and improvement during the trial period. The implantation procedure involves a small incision at midline back to feed the catheter to the appropriate level in the spine which will target the patient's specific pain. A second incision is made in order to place the medication reservoir and pump comfortably under the skin.

Complications of IT pump implants may be procedurally, or medication related [1]. Procedural complications can include infection, bleeding, severe headache, and catheter obstruction. Bleeding into the spinal column is a medical emergency and will require a visit to the nearest emergency room. Risks associated with medication are incorrect medication, pump reprogramming error and improper fill technique. Withdrawal symptoms may present with pump malfunctioning or programming error and severity of symptoms vary with class of medications. Withdrawal from morphine is unpleasant but not often life threatening [1].

Withdrawal from baclofen can be life threatening, thus patients are commonly given a prescription for oral baclofen to have available in-case if withdrawal symptoms occur. Patient will require pump refill every few months. The frequency of refills will depend on the patient use of the medication; the higher the usage, the more frequent the refills. Patients will also get a self-bolusing system to be able to bolus themselves at certain times in the day if needed.

Peripheral Nerve Stimulators

Peripheral Nerve Stimulation (PNS) was first described in the 1960s and now is commonly placed by pain physicians for pain relief. PNS is indicated when pain is confined to a specific distribution of a peripheral nerve, neuropathic pain, orofacial pain, trigeminal neuralgia, occipital neuralgia, hip pain, groin pain, post-thoracotomy syndrome, CRPS, post herpetic neuralgia, and more. It involves implanting a lead via needle along the desired nerve or area of pain to produce pain relief. Prior to implanting a PNS, a trial must be completed to confirm appropriate pain relief. The system can be operated with an implantable battery (as mentioned with SCS above) for certain brands or an external battery pack for other companies. Complications associated with PNS implants are lead migration, nerve injury, trauma, bleeding, infection and equipment failure [5].

Preoperative and Postoperative instructions for Spinal Cord Stimulators, Intrathecal Pumps, and Peripheral Nerve Stimulators

Pre-operatively, patients should follow similar anticoagulation guidelines as described with RFA and cryoablation. Please confirm with physician prior to stopping any anticoagulation. Patients will be sedated for the SCS and IT procedures, thus patients should follow the guidelines presented above under RFA and cryoablation. For PNS, sedation may or may not be used. This will need to be discussed with the physician at the appointment before the procedure.

Post-operatively, patients should follow same instructions as indicated with RFA and cryoablation as discussed above.

Patients will not be able to take showers or baths until follow up in one week [6,7]. It's recommended to take sponge baths in the meantime (instructions may vary among different physicians). Patients should check incision sites daily to monitor for infection, excessive swelling or bruising, redness or increased warmth and for fever over 100.4 F [6,7]. If they observe any of the listed issues, they should call their physician's clinic. Incision area should remain bandaged until follow up [6,7].

Patients will be given a back brace (only SCS and IT pump procedures) with instructions to limit bending, twisting or stretching of their body to prevent migration of leads. Patients should also limit raising their arms above their head for 1-2 weeks [6]. It is also recommended to limit driving as much as feasibly possible, although we understand the need to return to work and running errands. It's imperative to use caution when changing positions, for example it's recommended to log roll in and out of bed and to bend with knees [6,7]. Avoid lifting items weighing five pounds and straining during bowel movements [6,7].

Summary

We discussed in this chapter the most common advanced procedures in pain management but there are many other advanced procedures that can be discussed with treating physician on a case by case basis. There are new pain procedures every year, so conditions that we may not be able to treat today, may be treatable within the next few years.

References

1. Benzon, H. T. Essentials of pain medicine. Philadelphia, PA: Elsevier. 2018; 73(4) 663- 674

2. Narouze, S., et al. Interventional spine and pain procedures in patients on antiplatelet and anticoagulant medications: guidelines from the American Society of Regional Anesthesia and Pain Medicine, the European Society of Regional Anesthesia and Pain Therapy, the American Academy of pain Medicine, the international Neuromodulation Society, the north American Neuromodulation Society, and the world Institute of Pain. Regional anesthesia and pain medicine, 2015; 40(3), 182-212.

3. "Home Care after Cervical/Thoracic/Lumbar Rhizotomy (Radiofrequency)." University of Wisconsin Hospitals and Clinics, University of Wisconsin Pain Management Department, Aug. 2017, www.uwhealth.org/healthfacts/pain/5662.html

4. Mekhail, N., et al. Spinal Cord Stimulation 50 Years Later: Clinical Outcomes of Spinal Cord Stimulation Based on Randomized Clinical Trials—a Systematic Review. Regional anesthesia and pain medicine, 2018; 43(4), 391-406.

5. Trescot, A. M., et al. Peripheral nerve entrapments: clinical diagnosis and management. Springer, 2016.

6. "Home Care after Spinal Cord Stimulator Implant." University of Wisconsin Hospitals and Clinics, university of Wisconsin Pain Management Department, Aug. 2017, http://www.uwhealth.org/healthfacts/pain/6871.html

7. "Home Care after Spinal Cord Stimulator Trial." University of Wisconsin Hospitals and Clinics, University of Wisconsin Pain Management Department, Aug. 2017, www.uwhealth.org/healthfacts/pain/6805.html.

OPIOIDS AND THEIR HAZARDS

Introduction

Typically, when people think of pain medications, they think of opioids! There are likely many reasons for this notion varying from the drug class's history, government policy, public opinion, changes in medical practice, and most notably the current opioid epidemic which this country is facing. Whether we like it or not, opioids play a significant role in the treatment of pain, however, they are certainly not without their hazards and consequences.

For a drug class that has been around since the early 1800s, there is a surprising amount of confusion surrounding these medications and how to appropriately use them. One main reason is a lack of research-based evidence to support their use. Furthermore, when individuals discuss opioids, confusing terms such as opiates versus opioids, synthetic, natural, acute pain, and chronic pain are used. Misconceptions and misuse of terms often occurs due to this lack of knowledge. All of this leads to a harmful and potential deadly situation for patients and their families.

This chapter sets out to develop a better understanding of opioids for patients and their families. First, we will explore the history of opioids and our troubled relationship with them.

We will provide data regarding the use of opioids, describe their hazards, and provide statistics on the prevalence of negative outcomes. The hope is to describe why we as a society, and those in the medical profession, are so concerned with these medications. The second part of this chapter is to provide specific information about the drug class and different types of medication. Important terms will be defined to enhance comprehension. In addition, we will discover how opioids work at a basic level and the side effects associated with them. Finally, we will discuss each drug briefly in terms of their use in the treatment of chronic pain.

We will focus on how different drugs work, their unique concerns, and why one type may be chosen over another. As we alluded to earlier, opioids are a very complex and ever-changing topic. The hope is that with the following information we may be able to decrease some of the misconceptions and mystery surrounding chronic pain for patients and their families.

The History of Opioids

The word opioid is derived from the word opium. Opium is the dried remains of milky fluid extracted from poppy plants. Historic literature references opium-type substances as far back as 3400 B.C. in and around the Mediterranean [1]. Yet, the first opioid-type medication was not created until 1804 when German pharmacist Friedrich Serturner extracted morphine from opium. The drug was then marketed and sold for various ailments, but most notably as a pain medication. Serturner named the drug morphine after Morpheus, the Greek God of sleep, since after using the medication most patients tended to do so. Alarmingly, some fell asleep to such a degree that their bodies had troubling continuing to breathe. During some of his initial experiments Serturner almost killed himself and three children due to loss of consciousness and respiratory depression [2]. Thus, at their very introduction, opioids may have been demonstrating their hazards and providing us warnings.

Over the next 100 years many new opioids came to market including many of those we still commonly discuss today: heroin, codeine, and oxycodone. These drugs were unregulated until 1914 with the passage of the Harrison Narcotic Control Act in which the United States government first formally recognized the hazardous side effects of opioids, their addictive properties, and their abuse potential [3]. The government set formal standards for the medical utility of these medications and their availability. In the subsequent years an environment of generalized fear regarding opioids occurred.

Without large-scale evidence it was unclear how opioids should be prescribed and as a result, stigmas formed around their use. Even in cases such as cancer where there was likely a benefit, opioids were subject to extreme scrutiny. This is exemplified by the following comments made in the cancer pain literature of the 1950s, "every effort should be made to put off narcotic use until other measures have been exhausted... [and the patient's life] ... can be measured in weeks" [4,5]. We now know that cancer patients with severe pain may benefit from opioids earlier, not later, in their disease course. While the ideas expressed in the previous quote are quite extreme, they are important as it alludes to our current use of opioids as last line medications when other interventions have proved ineffective.

It wasn't until the end of the 20th century when opioid prescribing practices began to shift. During this time awareness regarding the undertreatment of pain started to be discussed in the medical literature. One of the first papers was published in a journal called the Annals of Internal Medicine in 1873. Two authors conducted 37 interviews with hospital patients who were prescribed opioids for pain and determined that over half of them were still experiencing moderate to severe pain [6]. This same message was echoed a decade later when two small chart reviews stated that the addiction rates for both hospitalized patients and chronic pain patients receiving opioids were rare [7,8]. At the time, there were limited medication options for the treatment of pain and these studies drew quite a deal of attention. Unfortunately, these studies were extremely small, less than 40 people, and used an inferior research method (i.e. not a double-blind randomized control trial). Thus, the initial spark for opioid use for non- cancer pain was minimal.

As we discussed in earlier chapters, the World Health Organization made a recommendation for prescribing opioids for patients with pain related to cancer in the late 1980s [9]. This was a major milestone that led to better treatment of pain in individuals with cancer. With the successes made in cancer pain management in the late 1980s and 90s, medical professionals began to wonder whether they had been undertreating all types of pain. Physicians began prescribing opioids and in particularly opioid/NSAIDs combinations for various disorders such as back pain, joint pain, and pain disorders. Thus, the use of opioids continues to spread from the world of cancer pain to chronic pain without any evidence-based justification.

This is no more apparent than discussions in the late 1990's when pain was described as "the fifth vital sign" [10]. While using "pain is the fifth vital sign" had noble intentions in bringing attention patients with acute and chronic pain, the phrase is also misleading. The word vital implies it is necessary for survival and that we could not live without it. However, the majority of people function every day without having any physical pain. It does not seem quite as vital as a heartbeat or regular breathing. Furthermore, if most chronic pain patients and their families were asked, we assume most of them would say they would prefer not to have pain.

Present day, the statistics, and the outcomes

Now that we have discussed the history, we need to discuss opioid use in the present day. In this section we will briefly discuss opioid use as it relates to chronic pain. We will summarize the current literature regarding outcomes and hopefully provide some insight into the current opioid epidemic and what is being done to reverse it.

According to the 2018 census date, it is estimated that approximately 11% of the adult population in the United States (36 million people) experiences chronic pain [11]. Of those patients, 3-4% are prescribed a long-term opioid [12]. Whereas there is strong research supporting short-term opioid use (up to 3 months), there is very little evidence supporting long- term effectiveness of opioids for treating chronic pain. [13]. What is equally troubling is that while many of these studies demonstrated the ability of opioids to help with pain short-term, they either did not assess or showed no improvement in patients' functionality overall. We all agree that controlling pain is important, however, an equally important goal is to assist patient in returning to a normal functional level to improve their quality of life.

There is also a difference between the evidence for using opioid pain medications and the amount that is currently being prescribed. For example, the United States reportedly consumes far more opioids per year than other countries even though there are a similar number of individuals suffering from pain [14]. The result has led to poor patient outcomes, misuse/abuse/diversion of medications, and most importantly, alarming rates of opioid overdose and death.

The cumulation of these problems has created what we commonly refer to as the "opioid epidemic". Following the increase in opioid prescribing in the 1990s, over 165,000 individuals died of overdose due to opioid-related pain medications in the United states from 1999-2014 [15]. During this same period, the number of individuals dying from illicit opioids such as heroin also increased, creating suspicion that when individuals ran out of their prescription drugs they were likely turning to illegal alternatives. Furthermore, it was reported in 2013 that almost 2 million people in the United States abused opioids or were dependent on their prescription opioid pain medication [15].

Currently, the large amount of extremely troubling data is driving the healthcare community and the government to change opioid policies to protect patients and their families. Many government agencies, both state and national, have passed laws guiding opioid prescribing. Further research is being conducted to analyze the problem, assess safety, and determine when and where opioids should be used. Most importantly, the opioid epidemic has demonstrated that close physician monitoring and a thorough discussion with patients and their family is crucial when prescribing opioid medications.

Definitions

Now that we have some perspective regarding the history of opioid medications and the current opioid epidemic, it is important to discuss some pertinent definitions. With the historical groundwork laid out, these definitions will likely have more meaning and will be easier to understand. It may be beneficial to even reread the previous section as it may provide further clarity in your understanding of the history of opioids.

To start, what is the definition of an opioid and how is it different from an opiate? An opioid is any substance that produces morphine-like effects by binding to special nerve receptors in the body aptly named the opioid receptors. These can be substances that occur in nature, such as extracts from the poppy plants, or substances created in labs.

Opioids which occur in nature are commonly referred to as non-synthetic or natural, whereas those created in a lab are referred to as synthetic. Or put even more simply, non- synthetic is extracted from nature and synthetic are man-made. Furthermore, some opioids are semi-synthetic which means they began as natural extracts but were altered in a lab from their original states. It is important to remember that not all things that are natural are necessary safe and beneficial.

Opiate, not to be confused with opioid, is a term used to describe only those substances that act like morphine and bind to an opioid receptor made in a lab. Thus, using our newly learned definitions opiates are a type of opioid that are synthetic (man-made). To differentiate, the word opioid, includes all medications that act like morphine both synthetic, semi-synthetic, and non- synthetic. Essentially opiates are a narrow definition of a subset of the drugs, where are opioids are a broad category of medications.

Another common term when discussing opioids is the word narcotic. It has many important historical ties including its use in our prior discussion of the Harrison Narcotic Control Act of 1914. If you search for this word on the internet, you will find many different definitions. The two most common definitions are vastly different. The first states that narcotics are substances that dull the senses and induce a profound sleep which can lead to mental status changes, stupor, or coma. Opioids easily fit within this definition, but so do other substances such as alcohol. The second definition states that narcotics are substances which are subject to restriction due to their side effects, medical utility, and addictive potential. Thus, this second definition includes a large group of substances such as alcohol, benzodiazepines and LSD. We believe that when discussing pain, the term narcotic should not be used due to the confusion it causes. We prefer precise descriptors such as simply using opioids or opiates when describing these medications.

General overview of how they work and common side effects

As we briefly discussed earlier in the chapter, opioids are medications that bind to special nerve receptors in the body cleverly named the opioid receptors. There are subgroups of opioid nerve receptors called Mu, Kappa, and Delta. These receptors are located all over a person's body and cause different effects depending on the type of receptor and its location. While binding to these opioid receptors provides their pain decreasing properties, otherwise known as analgesia, these medications also activate additional receptors which causes negative side effects. For instance, when opioids are ingested, they work their way into the bloodstream and to the brain where they may provide a patient pain relief. At the same time, they also bind to receptors that cause extreme sleepiness, lack of consciousness, and respiratory depression (slow and small breathing) which can be harmful to a patient's life. These are constant concerns of medical professionals when prescribing these medications, and sometimes these concerns are not stressed enough to patients and their families.

Other common side effects experienced by patients may include nausea, vomiting, constipation, small pupils, confusion, itchiness, urinary retention, lethargy, and seizures. The large variety of symptoms is due to the many different types and locations of opioid receptors throughout the body. The severity of these side effects depends on multiple factors such as the type of opioid, the dose prescribed, how long a person has been taking opioids, and their other health conditions. Conditions such as kidney and liver failure are especially impactful since most opioids are broken down by the liver and excreted by the kidney. When opioids are deemed necessary for treatment, a thorough conversation between the patient, the physician, and the patient's family is important since these medications have the potential to cause great distress and prevent individuals from functioning normally in their daily lives.

There are three important properties of opioids that may be commonly overlooked and not conveyed to patients. These are the risk of physical dependence, addiction, and hyperalgesia. All three of these properties are directly related to the dosage and length of time patients take opioid medications. For example, let's compare dependence, addiction, and hyperalgesia with caffeine, a more familiar substance. When people drink caffeine, they receive increased energy and focus. Over a long period of time their body becomes accustomed to the caffeine or even "craves" caffeine. If a person suddenly stops consuming caffeine they may begin to complain of headaches, feeling nauseated, or changes in mood. This is called physical dependence. It occurs when unpleasant physical symptoms occur after discontinuation of an addictive substance. When this occurs with opioids, people may have headaches, nausea, and mood swings similar to when you stop drinking caffeine, but they may also have more severe symptoms such as severe diarrhea, anxiety, cramping, and increased pain.

A common misconception is that physical dependence and addiction are the same thing.

Addiction is disease of the brain's reward and motivation processing which causes a person to utilize a substance even when they face substantial negative outcomes from its use. An example of addiction to caffeine is someone who continues to drink it despite life-threatening high blood pressure or trouble at work due to hyperactivity. In terms of opioids, addiction signs vastly vary but usually present with a negative social, economic, or health related outcome.

Thus, people with addiction can have physical dependence to a substance but at the same time cancer pain patients on opioids can have physical dependence but not be addicted. It is important to distinguish between addiction and dependence, as misunderstanding these two words may invite inappropriate stigmas.

The last side effect and one of the most challenging for patients and their families to understand is hyperalgesia. Hyperalgesia means increased and excess sensitivity to pain stimuli. Thus, opioids themselves can cause people to have more pain. Also, increasing opioid doses for these patients not only doesn't work, but will increase the patient's amount of pain. Think about it again in terms of caffeine. A person consumes caffeine to be awake and energized, but if they consume too much caffeine, they receive little or no benefit. They find themselves tired, possibly even more tired than they were without caffeine as the amount they are drinking each day begins to have negative effects. The same is true with opioids. Therefore, even prescribing opioids in the first place should be carefully considered; and if started, close monitoring and a discontinuation strategy are essential, even prior to the patient receiving the first dose.

Types of opioids

The last section will discuss commonly used opioid medications. We will focus on those frequently used for chronic pain but will also describe those that are used for acute pain, such as after surgery or after a trauma. Using opioids for acute pain is under the same scrutiny as using them for chronic pain due to limited evidence demonstrating benefit and a side effect profile that could lead to poor surgical outcomes (for example – severe constipation after abdominal surgery).

Opioids Used for Mild-Moderate Pain

Codeine

This non-synthetic opioid is less potent than morphine and is unique as it is broken down by the liver to form morphine itself. This oral medication is used for mild to moderate pain. Due to variation in patients' metabolism, some individuals may break down the medication too quickly or slowly. People who metabolize the drug too quickly are at risk for opioid toxicity (respiratory depression and death) and those who metabolize it too slowly, they may experience inadequate pain relief. While commonly found in cough suppressants and other pain medications, codeine is contraindicated for patient less than 18 years of age due to toxicity concerns.

Hydrocodone

Hydrocodone is another non-synthetic opium-derived medication which is available as a pill or oral liquid. It is also commonly used for mild to moderate pain since it is less potent than morphine or other oral opioids such as oxycodone. Hydrocodone pain-relieving effects usually last 4-6 hours. It is commonly combined with NSAIDs such as acetaminophen (Norco, Vicodin, Hycet) or with ibuprofen (Vicoprofen). These combined medications became popular in the late 20th century and are commonly employed for short courses after surgery. Of note, the combination of acetaminophen with hydrocodone (and several other opioids) has been responsible for many acetaminophen (Tylenol) overdoses which cause acute liver failure. Patients should always be certain that the total amount of acetaminophen they ingest per day is under the recommended three grams.

Oxycodone

Oxycodone is another oral pain medication that became popular when it was combined with other medications such as acetaminophen (Percocet), Aspirin (Percodan), and Ibuprofen (Combunox). Oxycodone is a semi-synthetic opioid that is 1.5 times more potent than oral morphine. Like codeine and other opioids, individuals differ in their ability to break down this medication, at times resulting in undertreatment of pain and at other times leading to opioid toxicity. Oxycodone also has multiple drug interaction with other medications metabolized by the liver such as antibiotics and anti-viral medications. This medication comes in both short- acting and extended-release formulations. Along with other opioids, oxycodone has led to issues with abuse and diversion (opioids used for non-medical purposes) during the opioid epidemic.

Tramadol

Tramadol (Ultram) is an extremely unique synthetic opioid that works in two separate ways. First, like other opioids, it binds weakly to opioid receptors and has effects similar to other opioids. In addition, Tramadol increase the amount of norepinephrine and serotonin, two neurotransmitters which have effects on pain and mood. This oral medication is weaker than oral morphine. Like codeine it has questionable utility in patients under 18 years of age. It is important to note that individuals considering this medication should be sure to tell their physician if they are on any anti-depressant medications as they could experience severe side effects.

Opioids used for Severe Pain

Morphine

As discussed previously, morphine was the first opioid created. All other opioid strengths are compared using morphine as the reference point. Morphine can be prescribed in oral, intravenous, rectal, and spinal formulations (epidural and intrathecal). Orally, morphine comes in both a short-acting and a sustained-release form (MS-Contin). Oral morphine takes longer to demonstrate effects compared to other opioids and the standard formulation usually lasts 4-5 hours. Like many of the opioids previously discussed, morphine may cause major problems in individuals with liver and kidney failure. Many of the metabolites (substances created by the breakdown) of opioids also bind to the opioid receptors.

Hydromorphone

Hydromorphone, also known as Dilaudid, is a strong synthetic opioid that is at least five times more potent than morphine. The usual duration of pain relief is 3-4 hours, but a sustained-release oral formulation now exists that lasts for longer periods of time. Like morphine, hydromorphone can be given in oral, intravenous, rectal, and spinal formulations. As with the next medication to be discussed, Fentanyl, the two medications are unique because their metabolites have very limited opioid properties. Thus, if they are not readily excreted by the body, they possess no significant side effects. Thus, these medications are better suited for individuals with kidney and liver impairment.

Fentanyl

Fentanyl is a synthetic opioid used for severe pain. This medication was originally created to be used for patients undergoing surgery and immediately post-operation. It is a fast- acting medication with a potency approximately 100 times more than morphine.

Fentanyl has no active metabolites which makes it an ideal drug in liver and kidney failure. Fentanyl comes in intravenous, transmucosal (through the lining of the mouth), spinal, and transdermal (skin) formulations. The transdermal patch is the only form used in chronic pain regimens and is primarily used for cancer pain, especially for those individuals who are not tolerating oral medications. A patch is applied to the skin and effects can last for up to 3-5 days until the patch needs to be removed and a new patch is applied. The patch application is not without challenges as the absorption of the medication can vary dramatically. Furthermore, the patch needs to be kept clean, dry, intact, and not exposed to heat such as a bath or hot tub as it can cause changes in the amount of drug released.

Methadone

Methadone is a long-acting opioid which is used for both chronic pain and opioid addiction. Its use in opioid addiction sometimes puts a negative societal stigma upon this medication. It has unique properties unlike any other opioid due to its long duration of action, difficulties in titrating to the right dose, high risk for overdose, and increased side effect profile including cardiac arrhythmias (abnormal heart rhythms). Individuals prescribed this medication often must undergo an electrocardiogram (monitoring of the heart) before initiation and every year following to screen for cardiac changes associated with arrhythmias. Before starting this medication, a thorough conversation between the patient, the prescribing physician, and the patient's family should be started in order to weigh the risk and benefits of the treatment.

Buprenorphine

Buprenorphine, like methadone, is a unique opioid since it can also be used in opioid addiction as well as for pain management. This semisynthetic opioid has a complex mechanism of action but is known to bind to certain opioid receptors only partially. It provides pain relief with less respiratory depression compared with other opioids. Furthermore, this medication blocks other opioids from binding to the opioid receptor and can deter individuals with addiction from taking other opioids it can be prescribed in oral, intravenous, and patch form.

Another medication, such as naloxone (an opioid blocking medication), can be added to buprenorphine to further prevent its misuse.

The Other Fentanyls

The remaining three medications which include sufentanil, alfentanil, and remifentanil are all synthetic fentanyl derivatives. These opioids are far more potent than morphine and have no clinic utility in chronic pain. They are all intravenous or spinal formulations and utilized by anesthesiologist in operative settings and would pose extreme danger outside these highly monitored settings.

Summary

It cannot be understated that the topic of opioid medication can be confusing and challenging. Whether we like it or not, opioids have played a significant role in the treatment of pain, but they are certainly not without their hazards, side effects, and consequences. As a class of medication, especially in the realm of cancer and chronic pain, we believe the World Health Organization Analgesic Ladder as discussed in the earlier chapters is currently the most logical way in prescribing these medications. It is vital for medical professionals, patients, and their families to have in-depth conversations regarding the risks and benefits of opioids. Hopefully through management of pain in a multimodal approach, we can continue to decrease the need for opioids and help decrease the negative effects it has on society in terms of the opioid epidemic.

Reference

1. Merlin, M. Archaeological Evidence for the Tradition of Psychoactive Plant Use in the Old World. Economic Botany. 2003;57 (3): 295–323

2. Sertürner F: Uber das Morphium, eine neue salzfähige Grundlage, und die Mekonsäure, als Hauptbestandtheile des Opiums. Annalen der Physik 1817; 5:56–75

3. Jones MR, Viswanath O, Peck J, Kaye AD, Gill JS, Simopoulos TT. A Brief History of the Opioid Epidemic and Strategies for Pain Medicine. Pain and Therapy. 2018;7(1):13-21.

4. Schiffrin MJ. The management of pain in cancer. St Louis: Year Book; 1956. pp. 7–8

5. Meldrum ML. A capsule history of pain management. JAMA. 2003;290(18):2470–2475.

6. Marks RM, Sachar EJ. Undertreatment of medical inpatients with narcotic analgesics. Ann Intern Med. 1973;78(2):173–81.

7. Porter J, Jick H. Addiction rare in patients treated with narcotics. N Engl J Med. 1980;302(2):123.

8. Portenoy RK, Foley KM. Chronic use of opioid analgesics in non-malignant pain: report of 38 cases. Pain. 1986;25(2):171–86.

9. WHO. Cancer pain relief. Geneva: WHO; 1986.

10. Campbell JN. APS 1995 presidential address. Pain Forum. 1996;1(5):85–8.

11. Nahin RL. Estimates of pain prevalence and severity in adults: United States, 2012. J Pain. 2015;16(8):769-780.

12. Boudreau D, et al. Trends in long-term opioid therapy for chronic non-cancer pain. Pharmacoepidemiol Drug Saf. 2009;18(12):1166-1175

13. Guideline for the use of chronic opioid therapy in chronic noncancer pain: evidence review. Amer. Pain Soc. http://americanpainsociety.org/uploads/education/guidelines/ chronic-opioid-therapy-cncp.pdf.

14. International Narcotics Control Board (2018). Narcotic Drugs Estimated World Requirements for 2018. United Nations Publication. https://www.incb.org/documents /Narcotic-Drugs/Technical-Publications/2017/.

15. Dowell D et al. CDC Guideline for Prescribing Opioids for Chronic Pain— United States, 2016. JAMA. 2016;315(15):1624–1645.

TREATING PSYCHOLOGICAL DISORDERS ASSOCIATED WITH CHRONIC PAIN

Introduction

When reflecting on the impact of chronic pain on one's life, it is easy to focus its multiple physical consequences. However, chronic pain's impacts are not only physical, with it impacting multiple other areas including mood, stress levels, physical abilities, sleep, social interactions, and ability to work. This change in the quality of one's life can unfortunately have a profound psychological impact, including heightened rates of depression, anxiety, and insomnia in people with chronic pain, as well as heightened emotional stress for their loved ones. Often times, these psychological impacts are overlooked by both the person with chronic pain and their treatment team, with much of the focus of treatment on obtaining physical relief. However, research is increasingly showing that psychological disorders associated with chronic pain can actually be associated with heightened pain, reduced success with pain treatment, poorer functioning, and reduced pain coping [1, 2]. Furthermore, effective treatment of these psychological symptoms, whether through medication [2] or psychotherapy [3] appears to not only reduce psychological distress, but also help to actually reduce an individual's pain and improve their pain coping.

There is even evidence that pain medications may be more effective in treating pain after psychological symptoms have been appropriately addressed [4]. Additionally, family members can benefit from additional support and treatment around their loved one's chronic pain [5]. With this in mind, this chapter focuses on normalizing the experience of psychological distress associating with chronic pain and discusses options for treatment to assist with this distress.

Depression

Depression and depressive symptoms represent the type of psychological distress most common in individuals with chronic pain. Studies show that up to 85% of individuals with chronic pain may struggle with significant depression symptoms. Individuals with multiple types of chronic pain or pain that has not yet been clearly diagnosed may be especially susceptible to this. There are a number of reasons that chronic pain may be associated with increased depression. For instance, living with chronic pain can be associated with the loss of activities that one used to enjoy and increased isolation from friends and family, both of which can make depression more likely. Interestingly, pain and depression appear to have a bidirectional relationship. In other words, while living with chronic pain may cause one to feel more depressed, the experience of depression can actually make pain worse, and can make pain a lot harder to deal with [6].

Despite depression being a common experience for individuals with chronic pain, there is evidence that it remains under-recognized by patients, their families, and their doctors. This is in part because people are often reluctant to discuss their emotions with loved ones or their medical team, despite the fact that most people with pain do struggle with increased stress, sad mood, or frustration at times. However, it also appears that the symptoms of depression are often missed in medical appointments. This is because depression does not only involve feeling sad or blue or being less interested in things that one used to enjoy (see next paragraph for more detail). It also involves symptoms like having low energy, sleep problems, or being less hungry than usual – symptoms that are typically associated with chronic pain, even when someone isn't depressed. As a result, depression can be missed, because it assumed that someone has lower energy or is sleeping worse simply because of their pain [6].

Depression may appear differently in different people. Symptoms to look out for include feeling more sad or blue than usual, being more easily frustrated, or feeling more emotional than usual. However, depression does not always mean being sad; it can also mean being *less* emotional, or "flat" and emotionally numb, and feeling less interested in things one used to enjoy. Depression can also be associated with feeling negative about oneself or one's abilities, and pessimism about the future. One may feel hopeless, helpless, or worthless, and one's self-esteem may be lower than usual. As mentioned above, depression can also affect how someone feels physically. People who are depressed may have sleep problems, which can be sleeping less or more than usual. They may feel very tired and fatigued, as well as lethargic, such that they feel like they are moving more slowly than normal. Sometimes the opposite can be true, such that a person feels agitated and restless, like they can't sit still. Individuals with depression may have an especially low appetite, such that they may even lose weight, or may eat more than usual and gain weight. Overall, depression is associated with a lot more difficulties than just feeling sad or being hard on oneself.

One of the most concerning symptoms of depression are thoughts of suicide. It is important to note, however, that just because someone has thoughts of dying does not mean that they are at risk of hurting themselves. A lot of people with depression or persistent pain find that they may fantasize about going to sleep and not waking up, largely due to a desire to escape from their current situation but are also clear that they would not take action to hurt themselves. However, suicide and suicide attempts are more common in individuals with chronic pain than in the general population [7], and thus thoughts of suicide should always be taken seriously in individuals with chronic pain. In particular, signs to look out for that suggest a risk of suicide include:

- Excessive sadness or moodiness, as often seen in depression.
- Sudden calmness. Oftentimes it is assumed that a sudden period of calmness is a sign that things are getting better, but it may actually be a sign that a person is feeling confident about the decision to harm themselves in the future.
- Increased isolation and withdrawal.
- Changes in personality and appearance.
- Increases in dangerous or reckless behavior.

- Making preparations to end one's life, such as writing a will or giving away personal belongings.

- Making statements or threats of suicide. While many people who hurt themselves do not make these threats, when they are made, they should be taken seriously.

If you are concerned about a loved one potential being suicidal, it can be worth it to ask them directly. There is a mistaken belief held by many that asking about suicide can trigger these ideas in people, whereas it can actually be relieving to have someone check in about these thoughts.

There is help out there for people struggling with depression and thoughts of suicide, whether seeking the appropriate mental health support (see below), speaking to a family doctor, medications, or even calling the National Suicide Prevention Lifeline (1-800-273-8255).

Getting help for depression is important for a number of reasons. First, depression can complicate the successful treatment of a pain condition. Pain rehabilitation takes a lot of time, energy, and effort. When depressed, it can be hard to motivate oneself to participate in rehabilitation, along with the other aspects of treating chronic pain that are so helpful, such as increasing activity levels, exercising, and seeking social support. There is also evidence that depression may cause people to be less tolerant of the pain that they do experience and feel more overwhelmed and discouraged by it. While treating depression may not necessarily get rid of one's pain, there is reason to believe that it does not only reduce pain levels but helps a person cope with their pain more effectively, feel less overwhelmed by it, and engage in other treatments and activities that help to better manage pain [1,2].

There is a number of psychological treatments shown to be effective in managing depression. The most widely known, and arguably most commonly practiced type of psychotherapy for depression is cognitive-behavioral therapy (CBT). This approach is based on the cognitive model, which indicates that an individual's response to a stressful situation is largely based on their thoughts about that situation. CBT typically focuses on teaching people to better recognize and challenge negative ways of thinking, as well as reduce unhelpful behavior patterns. Contrary to perceptions of psychotherapy involving years spent discussing family history and dreams while lying on the couch, CBT tends to focus on specific goals identified with the patient and is often time-limited, with considerable attention on practicing skills outside of sessions in the patient's daily life [8]. Adaptations of CBT have also been found to be beneficial for individuals with both chronic pain and depression. Mindfulness based cognitive therapy (MBCT) takes the basic principles of CBT and adds skills in mindfulness and stress management [9].

More generally, mindfulness training can be quite helpful in learning to better manage both depression and pain [9]. Mindfulness has been defined as "paying attention in a particular way: on purpose, in the present moment, and nonjudgmentally [10]". It can involve learning meditation skills, as well as ways of better responding to stress in the present moment. A number of programs and approaches have built on this concept and show significant evidence of benefits for coping with stress, medical issues, and depression, alongside a variety of other psychological stressors. For someone thinking about using mindfulness to help with their depression, consideration could be given to working with a psychotherapist skilled in mindfulness, attending a Mindfulness Based Stress Reduction group, participating in a local mindful meditation class, or reading one of several excellent books on the topic (see: *Wherever You Go, There You Are: Mindfulness Meditation in Everyday Life* by Jon Kabat-Zinn, *The Mindfulness Solution to Pain* by Jackie Gardner-Nix and Lucie Costin-Hall, or *The Mindful Way through Depression* by Mark Williams, John Teasdale, Zindel Segal and Jon Kabat-Zinn).

A number of other psychotherapies have been found helpful for depression. Acceptance and commitment therapy (ACT) can be especially beneficial when trying to cope with an unchangeable situation, such as a long-term chronic pain condition, diagnosis of a major medical issue, or a severe injury. As indicated by its name, ACT focuses on learning to accept and adapt to the "new normal" of certain medical restrictions, while still living a life that is meaningful. In contrast, interpersonal therapy (IPT) targets another challenging part of living with depression and chronic pain: its impact on your loved ones and interpersonal relationships. IPT focuses on improving social support and addressing problems in relationships. It can be used on its own, but also can be combined with CBT or mindfulness approaches in order to address a person's specific challenges [8].

Additionally, individuals struggling with depression may want to speak to their family doctor about an antidepressant. There can be a mistaken belief that because one's depression is a reaction to a stressful situation, namely living with chronic pain, that it is not treatable by medications that address brain chemistry. This has been shown to be untrue. Antidepressants can not only be helpful in reducing depression symptoms in chronic pain, but also can help to directly reduce the symptoms of chronic pain, even in those who are not depressed [11].

Anxiety

Anxiety can be a common experience in individuals with chronic pain, with some studies showing that as many as 70% of people with chronic pain report some anxiety symptoms [12], and anywhere from 10% to 62% of chronic pain patients can be diagnosed with an anxiety disorder [13]. There are a lot of reasons that anxiety and chronic pain may overlap. For one, stress tends to be heightened when dealing with a pain condition. Chronic pain can change many major life areas, including one's work, social life, and extracurricular activities, and it may be a struggle to figure out how to adapt. An individual may worry about the impact of their pain on their abilities in the future, or how to discuss their limitations with people who are used to them being healthy and able-bodied. Dealing with numerous medical appointments, awaiting test results, insurance issues, and medication side effects can be stressful. As such, it may come as no surprise that individuals with chronic pain may find themselves more worried and tenser than prior to their pain condition. Additionally, individuals with a history of anxiety prior to developing a pain condition may find that dealing with a pain condition exacerbates these symptoms.

Despite the fact that anxiety associated with chronic pain may seem reasonable, given increased stress levels, this does not mean that it should be simply accepted as a part of living with pain. Indeed, anxiety has been found across a variety of studies to worsen both pain symptoms and coping with these symptoms [2]. When stressed out, the human body goes through a series of physical changes, including increased muscle tension, heightened blood pressure, and shallow breathing, all of which typically exacerbate pain. Furthermore, when worried or feeling overwhelmed, it is easier to focus on one's pain and forget about helpful coping strategies. Many people fall into a vicious cycle with anxiety around their pain, such that they become so worried about their pain and the impact it may have on their life that they inadvertently make their pain worse. This is not to say, however, that their pain is *only* because they have stress; rather, many research studies have shown that most diagnosed pain conditions tend to worsen when stress and anxiety are not appropriately managed.

As mentioned above, some heightened stress or worry can be normal when dealing with the impact of chronic pain. However, there are some signs that additional support or coping skills may be helpful. This includes finding one's worries difficult to control, taking up large parts of their day, or result in sleep problems, irritability, muscle tension, or concentration difficulties. It is also worth seeking assistance for panic attacks. A panic attack is not simply feeling nervous or physically anxious, but rather going through a distinct period, typically lasting 20 to 30 minutes, of a number of overwhelming symptoms, which may include an increased heart rate, shortness of breath, trembling, nausea, dizziness, fear of dying, or fear of going crazy. It also becomes important to treat anxiety when it is starting to affect one's quality of life such as when one stops leaving the house due to fears or trying to avoid social activities.

The good news is that, similar to depression, there are a number of successful methods for getting help for anxiety. A large body of research indicates that relaxation training is particularly effective for reducing anxiety and pain symptoms [14, 15]. A variety of relaxation techniques can be used to assist with anxiety management, including breathing practice (e.g., diaphragmatic breathing, slowed breathing), autogenic training (which involves the repetition of suggestive phrases, such as "my shoulders are heavy and relaxed"), progressive muscle relaxation (which involves the tightening and relaxation of major muscle groups), and guided imagery (which involves imagining oneself in a safe and comfortable place, using all of one's senses). Relaxation training is available by meeting with a psychologist or other trained mental health professional, as well as through local meditation groups and centers, and a through variety of external resources, such as smartphone applications (e.g., Calm, Headspace) and books (e.g., *The Relaxation* and *Stress Reduction Handbook* by Martha Davis).

Mindfulness training, which was introduced in the above section on depression, has also been shown to be quite helpful for anxiety management [16]. Options for mindfulness training including working with a mental health professional skilled in mindfulness training, participating in a Mindfulness Based Stress Reduction group, connecting with a local mindfulness meditation class, reading a book on the topic (see above section on depression) or using online resources, whether paid (https://www.onlinecollegecourses.com/2012/11/25/9-great-mindfulness- courses-you-can-take-online/) or free (e.g., http://www.freemindfulness.org/download; https://palousemindfulness.com/).

CBT, which was introduced in the section on depression, has also been shown to be effective for the treatment of anxiety [17]. This type of treatment involves working with a psychotherapist to help better learn the impact of your behaviors and negative thinking patterns on your emotions and physical symptoms. One then makes gradual changes to the unhelpful behaviors, such as gradually facing feared situations, and learning to use evidence to challenge unhelpful worries. As with depression, this type of treatment tends to be shorter in duration and quite active in nature, such that a client works on "homework" between sessions to help generalize skills to their daily life. In addition to CBT, other therapeutic approaches, such as ACT (introduced above) which focuses on accepting what you cannot change while learning to live a meaningful life, also show success as another way of addressing anxiety [18].

While psychotherapy, mindfulness skills, and relaxation training all have considerable success in helping individuals struggling with anxiety and chronic pain, it may also be worth speaking to your family doctor about medications to help reduce your anxiety symptoms. There are also notable benefits to working on increasing physical activity, reducing caffeine, improving diet, and prioritizing sleep (see below) for anxiety management.

Insomnia

Insomnia is unfortunately a common difficulty for individuals with chronic pain. Estimates suggest that 60 to 80% of individuals with chronic pain have difficulties with falling or staying asleep. This may be due to challenges finding a comfortable position, pain causing awakenings throughout the night, pain being worse at night when there are fewer distractions, and the increased stress and worry that pain can cause. Unfortunately, pain and insomnia have what is known as a bidirectional relationship; in other words, pain can cause poor sleep, but poor sleep and associated fatigue can in turn cause worsened pain and more coping difficulties.

Complicating things further is that insomnia appears to be underreported and undertreated in chronic pain; patients will often focus more on their pain symptoms in the short time they have with their physicians and won't mention the struggles they are having with sleep [19].

However, the good news is that insomnia can be successfully treated without needing to over- rely on sedative medication; estimates suggest that 75% of cases can be treated by an informed and skilled treating provider. A large part of successful treatment involves correctly addressing the underlying issue that is causing the insomnia, rather than simply trying to treat the symptom. For instance, treating insomnia that is related to increased pain due to over-activity is different than insomnia related to worries about upcoming medical tests [19].

Insomnia can often be successfully treated by a focus on changing behaviors that are known to perpetuate poor sleep. This is known as sleep hygiene training and can make a tremendous difference in the sleep quality of individuals with chronic pain. However, it should be noted that work on sleep hygiene is rarely a quick fix. It can often take several weeks of consistent practice to break long-held habits that have made sleep worse; one should not be discouraged if they do not see dramatic improvements in sleep quality after a few nights of behavior changes. The American Sleep Association [20] provides a number of helpful guidelines, which include:

- Going to bed and waking at the same time whenever possible.
- Avoiding naps whenever possible.
- Getting out of bed when unable to sleep for more than 10 minutes at a time and do something relaxing and distracting.
- Only use your bed for sleep and sexual activity- do not hang out, read, or watch TV in your bedroom.

- Do not have your clock visible when trying to sleep.
- Avoid caffeine, alcohol, exercise, and food before bed.

However, for some people, sleep habit changes can be challenging to make without additional support or accountability or may not be sufficient on their own to improve sleep. Fortunately, there is also considerable evidence that CBT-I, a CBT treatment specifically for insomnia, can be of significant benefit [21]. It focuses not only on improving sleep hygiene, but also relaxation training and challenging negative thoughts that may contribute to one's insomnia. It is typically short-term in nature, often lasting around eight weeks. While meeting with a mental health professional trained in CBT-I can be especially helpful, there are also resources when this is not readily available, including books (e.g., *The Insomnia Workbook: A Comprehensive Guide to Getting the Sleep You Need* by Stephanie Silberman and Charles Morin; *Quiet your Mind and get to Sleep* by Colleen Carney, Rachel Manber and Richard Bootzin), websites (e.g., http://mysleepwell.ca), and online programs (https://www.sleepio.com/).

Family Members and Loved Ones

Much of the above discussion has centered on psychological struggles and symptoms that an individual with chronic pain go through. However, it is also common for family members and close friends to also experience an emotional impact of their loved one's chronic pain. It can be a struggle to see the one they love dealing with severe pain that they are unable to fix.

Oftentimes, their loved ones are unable to do the things they used to enjoy doing together, or may be struggling with depression, anxiety, or thoughts of suicide. Loved ones may have to pick up more of a financial role or do more around the house or for childcare. They may worry about what the future looks like for their loved one and their family. They may struggle with a steep learning curve around helping to manage a medical condition they know little about, as well as a lack of formal support and treatment, especially for those living in rural areas or with no health insurance.

Fortunately, there is information out there on how to best support a loved one with chronic pain. This includes educating oneself about the pain condition, helping keep their loved one accountable to medical recommendations, supporting them around exercise and seeking formal psychological support when necessary, and just being there to listen to the stress their loved one may be experiencing. However, there is less information available on managing caregiver burden. Caregiving for an individual with chronic pain can be associated with struggles with time management, increased stress, and feelings of loneliness. Research suggests that caregiving for someone with a chronic medical issue, while psychologically meaningful, can result in increased rates of depression, anxiety, and anger [22]. While it may be tempting for caregivers and loved ones to minimize distress in order to avoid upsetting the individual with chronic pain, it is crucial for their own well-being and the well-being of their loved ones to acknowledge when they are struggling and seek support as necessary. This may include joining an in-person or online support group for caregivers, delegating household tasks and learning to ask for help, or even being honest with friends and family about one's own emotional struggles. It may also be worth seeking more formal support, such as exploring a Mindfulness Based Stress Reduction group, looking into family or individual psychotherapy to help with adjustment to the "new normal" of life as a caregiver or loved one with chronic pain, or even reading about the issue (e.g., *When Someone you Love has a Chronic Illness* by Tamara McClintock Greenberg; *Surviving your Spouse's Chronic Illness* by Chris McGonigle). It is also important to remember that asking for help for when needed allows one to be a more effective and compassionate companion for your loved one.

Summary

Living with chronic pain is not only a physically challenging experience. It has impacts across all areas of one's life, including one's stress level, sleep, ability to participate in previously enjoyed activities, and interpersonal relationships. As a result of this, chronic pain is also a fundamentally emotionally distressing experience. It is not uncommon for individuals with chronic pain and their loved ones to struggle with increased depression, worry, physical anxiety, and sleep difficulties. Unfortunately, the psychological impact of chronic pain is not readily discussed in popular culture or medical settings, which can leave the many people who struggle with emotional distress feeling as though these difficulties are something unusual or shameful. It is important to realize that these symptoms are a normal part of adjusting to chronic pain, and in no way suggest that one's pain is any less real or valid. However, just because these symptoms are normal and common does not mean that an individual needs to learn to just live with them. Indeed, there are a number of effective options available to help to reduce emotional distress, worry, and sleep problems, from medications, to self-help options, to formal psychological treatment. Not only can these options help people with chronic pain and their loved ones to feel better psychologically-they can also help to reduce overall pain levels and improve pain management skills.

References

1. Rayner, L, et al. Depression in patients with chronic pain attending a specialized pain treatment center: Prevalence and impact on health care costs. Pain 2016; 157: 1472-1479.

2. Bair, MJ, et al. Depression and pain comorbidity: A literature review. Arch Intern Med 2013; 163: 2433-2445.

3. Morley, S, et al. Systematic review and meta-analysis of randomized controlled trials of cognitive behavior therapy and behavior therapy for chronic pain in adults, excluding headache. Pain 1999; 80: 1-13.

4. American Pain Society. Evidence shows benefits of psychological care in pain management. Retrieved from http://americanpainsociety.org/about-us/press-room/evidence-shows-benefits-of-psychological-care-in-pain-management.

5. Lewandowski, W, et al. Chronic pain and the family: Theory-driven treatment approaches. Issues Ment Health Nurs 2009; 28: 1019-1044.

6. Bair, MJ, et al. Depression and pain comorbidity: A literature review. Arch Intern Med 2003, 163; 2433-2445.

7. Tang, NKY, et al. Suicidality in chronic pain: A review of the prevalence, risk factors and psychological links. Psychol Med 2006; 36: 576-586.

8. Strunk, D. Depression. 2016. https://www.div12.org/psychological-treatments/disorders/depression/. Accessed 19 Sept 2017.

9. Kuyken, W, et al. Efficacy of mindfulness-based cognitive therapy in prevention of depressive relapse. JAMA Psychiatry 2016, 73; 565-574.

10. Kabat-Zinn, J. Wherever you go, there you are: Mindfulness meditation in everyday life. Hyperion Books, New York, 1994.

11. Khouzam, HR. Psychopharmacology of chronic pain: A focus on antidepressants and atypical antipsychotics. Postgrad Med 2016, 128: 323-330.

12. Castro MC, et al. Comorbid depression and anxiety symptoms in chronic pain patients and their impact on health-related quality of life. Arch Gen Psychiatry 2011; 38: 126-129.

13. Gatchel RJ, et al. Etiology of chronic pain and mental illness: How to assess both. Pract Pain Manag 2013; 11. Retrieved from https://www.practicalpainmanagement.com/pain/other/co-morbidities/etiology- chronic-pain-mental-illness-how-assess-both

14. Manzoni GM, et al. Relaxation training for anxiety: A ten-years' systematic review with meta-analysis. BMC Psychiatry 2008; 8: 41.

15. Schaffer, SD, et al. Relaxation and pain management. Am J Nurs 2004; 105: 75-82.

16. Hofmann SG, et al. The Effect of Mindfulness-Based Therapy on Anxiety and Depression: A Meta-Analytic Review. J Consult Clin Psychol 2010; 78: 169- 183.

17. Carpenter JK, et al. Cognitive behavioral therapy for anxiety and related disorders: A meta-analysis of randomized placebo-controlled trials. Depress Anxiety 2011; 35: 502-514.

18. A-Tjak, JG, et al. A meta-analysis of the efficacy of acceptance and commitment therapy for clinically relevant mental and physical health problems. Psychother Psychosom 2015; 84: 30-36.

19. Oliver RL, et al. Under-reported and under-treated, chronic insomnia coexists with - and perpetuates - chronic pain. Practical Pain Management 2002; 6. Retrieved from https://www.practicalpainmanagement.com/pain/other/co-morbidities/chronic-insomnia-pain.

20. American Sleep Association. Sleep hygiene tips. Retrieved from https://www.sleepassociation.org/about-sleep/sleep-hygiene-tips/.

21. Trauer JM, et al. Cognitive Behavioral Therapy for Chronic Insomnia: A Systematic Review and Meta-Analysis. Ann Intern Med 2015; 163: 191-204.

22. Rokach A, et al. Caregivers of chronic pain patients: Their loneliness and burden. Nursing and palliative care 2016; 1: 111-117.

PSYCHOLOGICAL APPROACHES FOR TREATING CHRONIC PAIN

Introduction

The International Association for the Study of Pain defines pain as "an unpleasant sensory and emotional experience associated with actual or potential tissue damage" [1]. The emotional experience of pain is something both patients and practitioners commonly overlook. Pain brings about changes in our mental and social abilities that augments its effects and duration. Chronic pain is an abnormal experience that brings about a great deal of stress, hardship, and mental anguish, not only for those who suffer from it, but for the patient's entire family and social support network. It is important to stress that chronic pain is something we as humans were not raised to or biologically designed to cope with.

Research has demonstrated that individuals with chronic pain suffer from increased rates of depression and anxiety [2]. Some studies have demonstrated depression rates as high as 80% in patients with chronic pain [3]. It is crucial for both patients and pain practitioners to be aware of these potential comorbidities and to realize that successful treatment of chronic pain requires concurrent treatment of a patient's mental and emotional wellbeing. Left untreated, patients underlying depression and anxiety can prevent adequate treatment response or worsen an individual's chronic pain.

There are many ways to treat depression and other psychiatric comorbidities associated with chronic pain including medications and intensive psychiatric counseling. This chapter resolves around psychoeducation and therapy-based approaches.

People often have preconceived notions when the words psychology, psychiatry, or therapy are used. Therapy-based approaches and the learning of coping mechanisms are research-based treatment strategies with proven benefits.

By understanding and utilizing certain psychological strategies, a patient and their family can treat pain, decrease its effects, reduce pain flares, and minimize its control over their daily life.

This chapter will begin by discussing the various coping mechanisms available for the treatment of chronic pain such as pacing strategies, relaxation strategies, and mindfulness. We will discuss the ideas behind each strategy and provide instructions for basic performance.

Then, more intricate psychological approaches for chronic pain such as cognitive-behavioral therapy, hypnosis, and biofeedback will be addressed. The goal of this chapter is to provide background knowledge and basic resources for patients and those who support them.

Hurt Versus Harm

Before diving into the multiple coping mechanisms for pain, it is extremely important to discuss the concept of hurt versus harm. This is a concept that many individuals, especially those who have suffered with chronic pain for months to years, find troubling and confusing. While pain is an unpleasant experience associated with actual or potential tissue damage, the same is not true for chronic pain. Chronic pain is pain that persists past normal healing. Chronic pain lacks the benefit of being an acute warning system for the body to tell an individual that potential or actual tissue damage is occurring [4]. This is the foundation of hurt versus harm. A person may experience pain or hurting, but no harm or tissue damage is occurring. It might be hard to imagine, but in some instances creating or working through some degree of acute pain may be necessary to recover from chronic pain.

Imagine a person who was told they should never run. They live their life walking from place to place, never picking up the pace, and never moving faster than needed. That person undergoes deconditioning as they have lost (or never gained) the appropriate fitness to perform an activity such as running. One day that same chronic walker watches a marathon on the television and decides that they want to become a runner. That person instantly jumps off the couch, walks outside, and begins to run as fast and as far as they can. Shortly after the person feels pain in their knees, ankles, muscles, and every other portion of their lower limbs. This new runner immediately thinks running cannot be good because it is painful! This is the exact problem when people misunderstand hurt versus harm as sometimes pain is a sign of growth and remodeling. Running is actually a very healthy activity. However, even if done correctly, it may cause pain. The pain experienced is a sign that the usually unused muscles are now being activated. The ligaments and bones have never been required to bear the forces of running and are now being compressed and worked. These changes may cause pain, but it's a good thing, as the runner's body is growing and strengthening to allow for this new activity. The muscle they build will help support them, allow them to run further and faster, and build even more muscle in the future without causing any harm.

This same concept can be related to an individual with chronic back pain who undergoes physical therapy. It may hurt in the beginning since that person is not accustomed to bending, stretching, and working their muscles due to their fear of pain. When they do start physical therapy, the pain they experience is not necessarily causing any harm. The strength and flexibility the person with chronic back pain gains can provide stability to their core and decrease the severity of pain.

With the new understanding that not all pain is harmful and endurance of a short degree of pain may be beneficial in treating chronic pain, one might ask themselves the logical question, "How can I get through this pain?" The following sections list multiple coping strategies to decrease the effect of pain. Each strategy may not work for everyone since coping is not a "one size fits all" option. The following list has been utilized by individuals with chronic pain with great deals of success in the past.

Coping Strategies in Pain

Goal Setting

One of the first strategies in enduring chronic pain is goal setting. This strategy may also be one of the hardest as it is based on a person's self-motivation. For individuals with chronic pain it is important to determine which activities improve their quality of life. These activities may range from as simple as playing with grandchildren or taking daily walks in the park with friends to something more difficult such as running a race or continuing their active job. The goals must be set based on what is important to each person and on their ability to obtain them.

For goal setting to be a positive solution for patients with chronic pain we believe it is important to base a framework around a goal. First, the patient needs to identify a functional goal. For example, let's use the goal of walking in the park with friends as a goal for a patient with chronic back pain. The second step would be to determine the challenges faced when setting such a goal. For a chronic back pain patient, it may be that walking in the park causes their back pain to worsen. Worsening chronic pain is major challenge, but it is one that can be overcome using therapy strategies. The third step in goal setting is to identify what the person is willing to give up reaching their goal. In this example, the person may be willing to give up a few hours a week to participate in physical therapy or they may choose to push themselves walking further or more often knowing that their pain will be slightly worse and preparing for it. Framing goal setting in those three steps, 1) what is my goal, 2) what are the challenges preventing my goal, and 3) what will I have to sacrifice to achieve my goal can make it easier to get started and to reach a positive outcome.

Pacing Strategy

Pacing strategy is another method of coping with chronic pain that can be used very easily within the context of goal setting. Pacing involves setting a series of small challenges or goals over a course of time which allows a person to slowly build up to a larger goal. Prior studies have demonstrated that using pacing strategies in combination with goal setting is effective in improving outcomes in patients [5].

If we refer to our example of the chronic back pain patient who would like to walk in the park with their friends, we can show how a pacing strategy can be used to reach this goal. Let say the patient's friends usually walk a mile in the park each day. Initially this may be an insurmountable goal for the patient. However, if the large goal is split into smaller goals then reaching the goal may become more realistic. An example pacing strategy would be to walk a quarter of a mile each day for one week, then add a quarter mile to their walk each week until they can walk the full mile. Failures can be expected along the way but will likely be fewer as the patient is able to achieve each smaller goal.

Social support

It is extremely important for individuals with chronic pain to own their illness for two reasons. First, individuals may internalize their symptoms or the related stress, leading to negative outcomes not only for the individual, but also their friends, family, or coworkers.

Changes in a person's behavior, due to chronic pain, are often incorrectly interpreted by those around them and can lead to severe negative perceptions. Social support is another coping strategy that is very effective if used in accompaniment with the prior two strategies goal setting and pacing. If a person has family and friends around them that know their goals, they can help motivate the individual to reach them. They can help inspire positive ideas and enforce positive actions almost like a motivational coach. In our back-pain example, the patient could have a family member walk with them each day as they work up to their goal distance of one-mile distance. The loved one is there to provide positive reinforcement, motivate, and make working on the goal more enjoyable.

Self-Guided Cognitive Techniques

Other coping mechanisms that are beneficial in treating chronic pain are self-guided cognitive techniques. These strategies revolve around the individual suffering from chronic pain to become their own positive motivating force. They complete these goals by using self-talk, challenging negative thoughts, and decreasing the focus on their pain.

Self-talk, as the name implies, is either internally or verbally talking through the pain.

This may be used when exercising or attempting goal challenges but can also be applied during pain flares. It helps to rationalize one's personal pain symptoms. For example, the patient may state to themselves, "I realize this pain is intense, but it will not last", or even, "a little pain now while working out will decrease a lot of pain later." By utilizing self-talking, the person becomes their own coach.

Challenging negative thoughts is another effective cognitive strategy. Everyone has times in their life when they feel down or sad. In patients with chronic pain, many of these instances may be brought on by the pain itself or by the repercussions of pain. During these times it is easy to let negative thoughts change our mood or self-worth. By identifying these negative thoughts and challenges for ourselves, we can make major strides in decreasing pain. The goal is for patients to realize that they do not have to let the pain define their life.

Another self-cognitive strategy to improve outcomes in chronic pain is decreasing one's focus on it. As alluded to in the prior paragraph, when a patient dwells on negative thoughts, the thoughts likely worsen. The same can be said when a person dwells on their chronic pain and fails to work through it; the pain can begin to define them and their existence.

When negative thoughts occur, or when a person experiences a pain flare there are ways to decrease their focus on the pain. It is understandable that when pain and a depressed mood are at their worst, individuals cannot perform their normal activities, but this does not mean they should sit around and dwell on it. Even though the pain may be severe there is often something enjoyable the patient can do even while they are experiencing it. For patients with back pain or peripheral neuropathy, swimming or warm water aerobics may be soothing. Those individuals may not be able to go on long walks or complete more demanding tasks when their pain is at its worse, but instead of focusing on the negatives they can enjoy a more productive and relaxing activity. These activities can improve the patient's pain and mood acutely and increase their functionality over the long term.

Breathing, Imagery, Distraction

There are various other coping strategies to help patients with unremitting pain. Some of these have been previously discussed or will be discussed in later sections. For the sake of completeness, we will discuss several of these techniques before we proceed.

Guided breathing is a strategy many people utilize to mentally work through acute pain attacks. Simply taking slow deep breaths and focusing on bringing air in and out of their lungs allows a patient's body and mind to relax when pain is at its worse. It allows a patient to gain their composure and work through the pain both mentally and physically.

Imagery is also a great strategy for coping with acute pain. Picturing yourself at your favorite vacation destination or doing an activity you enjoy without pain can be very powerful. It can also help completely alleviate pain for certain people. Again, these types of activities allow an individual to relax tense musculature and to decrease stress during and after pain flares.

We touched on distraction earlier when we discussed decreasing pain focus. Distraction is a very effective coping strategy when facing pain. If we distract our minds and our bodies with an activity we enjoy, we do not dwell on the pain. This may be as simple as performing your daily job which you love or playing piano/any similar activities. Each person should have activities they enjoy doing! The patient may still have pain while performing the activity, but it can be overcome by their passion and love for the task at hand.

Other Active Coping Strategies

As we have seen thus far many of the previously discussed strategies are very thorough in their processes for facing pain. There are also very simple active coping strategies that people commonly overlook. Some of these active strategies may be things they already do but do not realize such as trust and education. Trusting in divine help in response to disease can have a major impact. For example, trusting that God will help or praying to become healthy may be useful. In general trusting in a higher power to help improve a disease can allow people to overcome pain/stress. Also, simply trusting in the medical help a person is receiving from health care providers is important. This means believing in the treatments you are receiving from interventions to prescribed medications. Just knowing you have ways to decrease the burden from pain is useful, but commonly overlooked. Those suffering from chronic pain should also cope by searching for more information and alternative care. You can never be too educated on pain or illness. Becoming properly informed, finding external sources about a disease, and discovering ways to become healthy again are great coping strategies.

Another simple strategy that is easy to employ is having a conscious way of living. This includes cognitive and behavioral strategies such as healthy diet, physical fitness, and living a healthy life style. Also, having a positive attitude is important. Focusing on positive thinking, realization of dreams/wishes, and avoiding thought about illness can help draw your attention away from pain and towards things that improve quality of life. Pain can also serve as a reason for reappraisal. In using reappraisal, you see an illness or pain as a chance to think about what is essential in life. The pain becomes a reason to determine life's meaning and determine how being in pain affects you. In conducting these reappraisals, you may develop a greater appreciation of life and what you will continue to do to make life great regardless of the pain.

As we have discussed so far in this chapter there are many ways that individuals with chronic pain can help themselves. Patients who suffer from pain must set goals in their lives, like the rest of us. These goals may be harder to obtain due to pain, but most are still achievable. Through use of pacing strategies and enrolling social support one can overcome challenges, decrease their pain, and improve functionality. Furthermore, using the self-guided cognitive strategies and various other techniques may help the patient take control of their situation and become their best weapon for decreasing chronic pain and the negative thoughts that sometimes come with it.

Psychological Approaches for Chronic Pain

The next portion of this chapter will shift from the less formal coping strategies to advanced psychological approaches used for the treatment of pain. Most of these strategies are proven to be of significant benefit in the chronic pain population. We briefly discuss each and provide some examples for their use.

Cognitive-Behavior Therapy

Cognitive-behavior therapy was first developed in the 1970s to treat depression, but it has also been used in those individuals suffering from chronic pain [6]. The basis of cognitive behavior therapy is improving functionality by focusing on gradually overcoming a person's fear of activities that trigger pain. It also involves introducing healthy habits.

This approach also focuses on overcoming two other aspects of the chronic pain experience: catastrophizing and kinesiophobia. Catastrophizing is when the person tends to magnify and dwell on pain experiences. Kinesiophobia is the fear of pain as a sign of serious bodily harm [7].

Cognitive behavior therapy uses graded exposure and relaxation techniques. Graded exposure is when a person is repeatedly introduced to a situation for which they are uncomfortable or fearful. This is completed slowly but briefly the first time, and then continually increased in both frequency and duration until the person is no longer fearful. An example of cognitive behavior therapy use in chronic pain would be a person with neck pain who refuses to move their neck due to fear of pain. The person wears a neck brace continuously which weakens their neck muscles and augments their pain. Through using cognitive-behavior therapy the individual may initially remove the collar for a short period of time, possibly as short as 5 minutes. The time without the collar would be then extended: 10 minutes, 1 hour, 1 day, 1 week, until the patient no longer needs it. Once the patient is comfortable without the neck brace, they can start adding on neck stretches. Again, this process would be slow. First the patient would start with only a couple of stretches, then maybe ten stretches, increasing each time until they were back at normal functionality and pain free. It is the summation of many small victories that achieves the final goal.

During this time the patient may have constant fears that they are doing severe damage (kinesiophobia). They should be coached through the fear or taught relaxation techniques to overcome their fears. The relaxation techniques serve a secondary function as they may also directly help the painful symptoms and reduce the stress surrounding their chronic pain. This multi-focused approach is one of the reasons cognitive behavior therapy has a large degree of successful utilization in chronic pain patients.

Mindfulness-Based Therapy

Mindfulness therapy works by bringing a patient's attention to experiences occurring in the present moment. Like cognitive behavior therapy, this concept has its roots back to the 1970s and has been demonstrated to be effective by many high-quality studies. For individuals with chronic pain, mindfulness therapy can bring self-attention to other sensations that the body is experiencing, while ignoring the sensations of pain.

The practice of mindfulness therapy can take place anywhere. A routinely employed method is to sit down on the floor or in a chair, close one's eyes, and simply pay attention to natural breathing. In doing so, the person does not need to control or change their breathing, but simply observes it. They feel the air move from their lungs, through the airways, out their nostrils, and back again. Individuals can undergo this process at set times throughout the day or whenever pain becomes intense. They should focus solely on the sounds, sensations, and actions of their body throughout this time. If their mind wanders, they should regain their focus in a non-punitive way [8].

Another commonly utilized form of mindfulness is that of tactile sensation. Rubbing an object such as a soft pillow or velvet cloth may be useful. Instead of focusing on the pain, the patient should focus deeply on the texture of the object. They focus on the warmth, the elasticity, or the coarse edges of the object while decreasing their attention on their anxiety or discomfort. Again, the therapy should be based on moment-by-moment awareness of feelings, body sensations, and the surrounding environment through ideas of acceptance and understanding, not control.

Biofeedback

Biofeedback is a hot topic in pain currently and a modality that is highly effective for treating chronic pain. Just as with the other techniques discussed, biofeedback is not a pain cure, but rather a method of reducing its burden both mentally and physically. Biofeedback can be easily understood if you break down its name into its root words. "Bio" refers to one's body, whereas "feedback" means processing the information the body provides us. With training and the use of tools such as mirrors or instruments, a patient can take control of their pain or other aspects of their body. Biofeedback can also be used to control functions of a patient's body of which they may not even be aware such as heart rate or even body temperature.

As a warning, biofeedback may require special devices and more advanced training by a psychological practitioner to get started, but it is something that can easily be recreated by a patient at home. Biofeedback is usually performed in a series of steps. First, the patient and/or practitioner determines the factors related to the patient's pain and identifies how a person reacts the pain. If the patient has chronic hip pain, they may tense the painful leg, hurting, stress out, and raise their heart rate which worsens the pain, alters body mechanics, and causes disruption in their life. The second step is to identify a physical response that a person can focus on and control. For this example, it may be heart rate or muscle tension. A therapist can teach a patient strategies to decrease their heart rate or muscle tension. These results can be monitored with a heart monitor or electromyography to assess effectiveness. The last step is simply for the patient to identify the triggers themselves and utilize the tools to complete the exercises on their own.

Hypnosis

When many people think of hypnosis, they think of a someone swinging a watch in front of their face telling them they are going to get very sleepy until they are under their control. This is far from how hypnosis is used in treating pain. Hypnosis uses both the power of suggestion from either another person or from the individual dealing with their pain. It is clinically effective for several different types of chronic pain including low back pain, cancer pain, and fibromyalgia [9]. Furthermore, hypnosis can be learned very easily by a person with chronic pain or a family member. Its effect can be used daily for confronting chronic pain, breaking up the cycle of pain, or simply working through a pain flare.

The goal for hypnosis, like mindfulness therapy, is to focus a person mind [9]. Upon initiation of hypnosis, the patient focuses on a word, phrase, or activity that comforts them such as breathing, dreaming about laying on a beach, or even repeating a word such as "relax". The goal is to center one's mind on a single entity and eliminate all other distractions including the pain. Once the patient's mind is focused, they can slowly introduce positive thoughts that improve mood and provide self-worth.

If the patient has difficulty relaxing while attempting hypnosis, he/she can also use progressive muscle relaxation or autogenic training. To use progressive muscle relaxation the patient begins to focus on relaxing the body slowly one muscle at a time. For instance, if the patient experiences neck pain, they may start focusing on relaxing the arms in a neutral position, then their shoulders, until finally reaching the neck. In autogenic training the person can use guided imagery or body awareness to overcome stress or anxiety. The patient gets into a comfortable position and focuses on the heaviness of a body part or imagines their painful area being slowly massaged in a pleasant manner. Again, the idea is to overcome the negative aspects of pain such as depression, anxiety, or stress via controlling the patient's focus and suggesting to the mind that it is not as bad or not occurring at all.

Acceptance

Acceptance, though not truly a psychological approach is an important concept that should be discussed along with chronic pain. To various degrees, certain conditions such as diabetic peripheral neuropathy, failed back surgical syndrome, or fibromyalgia may not have complete cures. There are treatments available to help improve these chronic pain conditions but not eliminate them. Commonly, patients with chronic pain grasp at any hope that they may one-day return to being pain free. While it is important to recognize this idea, it is also extremely important for pain practitioners to tell patient when this goal may be out of reach and set goals that are obtainable. Certain patients can understand that they may always have pain and they are able to accept that concept.

Those individuals realize that no matter what they do they will likely live with some degree of pain for the rest of their lives. They make goals to remain active, live healthy lifestyles, and do all they can to minimize the impact their pain has on their life. Many of these patients can live happy and productive lives, possibly even more than individuals who do not suffer from chronic pain. These people with chronic pain may face hardships no person should have to bear but remain productive members of society, which is no small feat. It is an accomplishment that should be respected and praised.

Summary

Pain is an unpleasant sensory and emotional experience associated with actual or potential tissue damage. The emotional experience of individuals who suffer from chronic pain should never be overlooked. Through this chapter, we have discovered that there are many individual coping strategies and psychological approaches to enhance one's mood and pain experience. These treatment strategies are as important as medication, physical therapy, and interventions. They should be routinely offered by pain practitioners and asked requested by patients with every encounter.

Reference

1. Bonica, J. J. "The need of a taxonomy." Pain 6 1979; 247-248.

2. Gatchel, R. "The biopsychosocial approach to chronic pain: scientific advances and future directions." Psychological bulletin 2007; 133.4: 581.

3. Bair, M., et al. "Depression and pain comorbidity: a literature review." Archives of internal medicine 2003; 2433-2445.

4. Treede, Rolf-Detlef, et al. "A classification of chronic pain for ICD-11." Pain 2015; 1003.

5. Bodenheimer, Thomas, and Margaret A. Handley. "Goal-setting for behavior change in primary care: an exploration and status report." Patient education and counseling 2009; 174-180.

6. Butler, AC, et al. The empirical status of cognitive- behavioral therapy: A review of meta-analyses. Clin Psychol Rev 2006; 26: 17-31.

7. Buenaver LF, et al. Cognitive behavioral therapy for chronic pain. In Fishman SM, Ballantyne JC, Rathmell JP, (Ed), Bonica's Management of Pain 2010; 1220-1230.

8. Creswell, D. "Mindfulness interventions." Annual review of psychology (2017): 491-516.

9. Elkins, Gary, et al. "Hypnotherapy for the management of chronic pain." Intl. Journal of Clinical and Experimental Hypnosis (2007): 275-287.

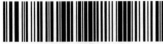
62113146R00098

Made in the USA
Columbia, SC
29 June 2019